Diverticulitis Cookbook 2021

Detailed 3-Phase Diet Guide with More Than 200 Easy & Delicious Diverticulitis Recipes with Easy to Find Ingredients. 21 Day Meal Plan & Index Included.

Author: Sophia Robinson

Table of Contents

Introduction

If you've been diagnosed with diverticular disease, you may be feeling uncertain about the future and what you can and can't eat. You're probably already aware that your diet will have a big impact on the severity of this disease, but what should you consume or avoid? This book is going to help you with that. The diverticulitis diet is one which many people who suffer from diverticular disease turn to as a means of managing the disease and minimizing the attacks. It can help to make life more comfortable, and it is not as restrictive as many diets you may come across. If you suffer from diverticular disease, you may find it is a great way to manage your condition. The diet is mostly focused on trying to include more fiber in your everyday meals, and cutting back on fiber when you are in pain. A high fiber diet reduces your risk of developing diverticular disease in the first place, as does making sure you are hydrated. While a diverticulitis diet is not a replacement for medical treatment of this condition, it may help you to control it and reduce the symptoms associated with it.

Diverticular disease is contributed to by various factors, but it is thought that you are more at risk if you eat a lot of animal protein, you're obese, or you're a heavy smoker. So, what should you eat if you are following a diverticulitis diet? How do you get that fiber boost you need?

What you should eat depends on whether you are having a flare-up or not at the moment. If the polyps in your gut have become inflamed or infected by something, you are probably in pain, and you may struggle to eat or digest food properly. If the polyps are not currently inflamed (diverticulosis), you can eat normally, and you should make the most of this situation to minimize your risk of diverticulitis. So, let's explore the two different options – what to eat when you're suffering, and what to eat when things feel fine to you. Note that this section will cover the general rules, with a few suggestions of the specific foods you should select. For a more complete list of suggested foods, see the section on Approved Diverticulitis Foods, which is full of ideas about things that you can eat.

Foods To Include During Diverticulosis

So, what do you want to eat when you have diverticular disease, but you are not suffering from any symptoms at the moment? Lots of fiber is the first answer, because fiber helps to keep things moving in your guts. This reduces the pressure on your colon and your risk of constipation – something that often contributes to the development of this disease in the first place. Including plenty of fiber, drinking lots of water, and exercising thoroughly is the best way to keep yourself healthy when you aren't enduring a flare-up.

What should you include?

Lots of fruits and vegetables, particularly high-fiber options like strawberries and bananas. These are soft foods that will keep your guts moving well. You may also want to add things like prunes to your regular diet.

Legumes are good for you too, and they make a nice alternative to meat if you are trying to reduce your meat consumption (cutting out red meat is particularly good for this kind of diet). Swap mince for lentils to create a satisfying meat-free lasagna, or add beans to your meals to bulk them out and help yourself feel full without meat. Nuts are also fine, contrary to popular belief; they are broken down thoroughly by the body and don't contribute to constipation or pressure on the guts.

Whole grains are a further good option, so swap white bread for wholegrain bread, and try out wholegrain pasta, too. Brown rice instead of white is also better for you, so try this as an alternative. The extra roughage and fiber should help to keep your digestive system functioning well, and the fiber helps to draw more water into your digestive system.

Foods to Include When Symptoms Begin

If you are starting to suffer from some of the common symptoms of diverticular disease, you may wish to reduce the amount of fiber that you consume. Cut back on whole grains, and reduce the amount of fiber you are eating each day.

Do keep drinking plenty, as water will help to ease pressure on your digestive system. Keep eating well, but don't try to pack as much fiber into your diet.

Foods to Include During A Flare-Up

When you're suffering from a flare-up, you want to reduce the amount of fiber in your gut. You need to minimize the pressure on your digestive system, and that means reducing fiber or indeed all food. Often, people suffering from a flare-up of diverticulitis eat very little until the episode has passed.

You should speak to your doctor when you're in pain, because they may recommend that you move to a clear liquid diet for a while, allowing the irritation to subside and taking the pressure off your digestive system.

A clear liquid diet includes things like pulp-free juices (e.g. apple), clear broths, water, and Jell-O. It doesn't count soup, so don't eat this. If you are on this sort of diet, you need to rest lots and avoid anything strenuous, as you may be prone to faintness and lacking in energy. This sort of diet shouldn't be followed for longer than a doctor suggests.

Alternatively, your doctor might just tell you to switch to a low-fiber diet if the flare-up is not so severe. In this case, you can continue to eat normal food, but you should swap your whole-grains for the white alternatives (bread, pasta, rice). You can eat potatoes, but these should be peeled, and all protein consumed should be very tender, such as shredded chicken, baked fish, and eggs.

Don't eat heavy foods or Large portions for a while, and discuss any concerns you have with your doctor before you continue to eat that food.

Reduce your fruit intake, staying away from high-fiber fruits and particularly the skins, which contain insoluble fiber that will irritate the gut. Instead, opt for canned fruits and soft options such as melon. Pair these with other high-protein, low-fiber options such as Greek yogurt and cottage cheese, or milk. These are soft foods that will give your body the nutrients it needs without worsening the inflammation.

Careful management will help you to overcome an episode of diverticulitis, but it is important to think about what you are eating and avoid foods that will further irritate your guts, or you could make both the pain and the polyp inflammation worse. Reduce the strain on your digestive system, and you should hopefully find that you recover more quickly, and the episode is less severe.

Gain an Understanding of Fiber and How It Affects Your Gut

So, why all the fuss about fiber?

Doctors that specialized in digestive tract illnesses have looked at what most people eat as a daily part of their diet and found that it is lacking in many of the essential nutrients that people should be eating for excellent digestive health.

One of these ingredients is a diet that is much higher in fiber than is previously prescribed. One of the major contributors to the development of diverticulitis is that a person has difficulty in passing waste out of the colon through the rectum.

A diet high in fiber will make this much easier and alleviate much of the problem. After the muscles in a person's colon spend years straining to perform their function due to a diet that is low in fiber there is a development of this issue. Particularly in the United States this can be seen. Doctors start to realize that the colon is becoming a bit stretched which makes it even more difficult to pass excrement from the body and the stool needs to be even bulkier to be moved out without difficulty.

There was a study done by the Journal of Nutrition that observed nearly 45,000 health professionals participating in a long-term study. They learned that when a person ate a diet that was high in fiber, they lowered the risk of contracting Diverticular disease by somewhere in the neighborhood of 40%.

A high fiber diet presents a lot of other benefits as well. It fills your stomach easily and suppresses your appetite which can majorly in losing weight. Losing weight can help fight against developing Diverticular disease indirectly. Diverticular disease is much more likely to put a woman in the hospital if she is overweight or inactive. This is according to a study that was published in the American Journal of Gastroenterology.

It is recommended currently that ¾ ounce of fiber should be consumed by women each and every day, while men should eat even more fiber, being advised to try to consume about 1½ ounces of fiber in the daily diet. Even with these warnings the average American eats about ½ ounce of fiber – a woefully low portion. One of the best ways to augment your lack of fiber is to include foods that are high in fiber at every meal and also for snacks throughout the day.

Great sources of fiber for your diet include whole grains, oatmeal, whole wheat bread, and barley. There are also some other great foods that you can dig into like lentils, fruits, vegetables and beans to give your diet a kick. One of the best snacking foods for a fiber input into your diet is to eat plenty of dried fruits which are a terrific source of fiber. This type of eating plan is referred to as a whole foods diet because it includes a lot of foods that are not processed and treated with chemicals like white rice and white bread.

Both of these are going to help cause diverticulitis rather than cure it. Eliminating the food that is bad for you is just as important as adding the food that is good for the body. There are two types of fiber to consider: soluble and insoluble. They are both an important part of a healthy diet but for different reasons. The insoluble fiber that is found in vegetable peels of fruit and seeds will add bulk to the stool in the colon and make it easier to pass reducing the wearing strain on the muscle. Soluble fiber is the other kind that a body needs, and it comes from foods like oatmeal, barley, and many Fresh fruits like apples. This adds to the moisture located in the stool and that makes it easier to pass through the colon and reduces the strain.

The recommended intake of fiber is generally:
- Women age 19 to 50 = 25 grams per day
- Women age 50+ = 21 grams per day
- Men age 19 to 50 = 38 grams per day
- Men age 50+ = 30 grams per day

Please contact your doctor to confirm that these values are okay for your specific scenario.

Drink More Fluids

Many overlook the importance of staying hydrated, but this tip may be the most effective in maintaining gut health. Drinking more fluids can help a high fiber diet be moved even easier through the digestive process with fewer chances of obstructions developing. Keeping the fluid intake into a normal level is all that is needed. There doesn't seem to be much of a benefit for drinking excessive liquids during the day. Look to drink as many non-calorie beverages as you can with your diet each day that means no limits to water or tea.

The recommended water intake is generally:
- Men age 19+ = 12 cups (about 3 liters) per day
- Women age 19+ = 9 cups (about 2 liters) per day

Please contact your doctor to confirm that these values are okay for your specific scenario.

The Latest Scientific Research on the Diverticulitis Diet

Research in this field is limited, and there are surprisingly low levels of awareness about the disease, in spite of how common it has become. Around 50% of Western adults over 50 are at risk of the disease, and that rises to 75% at age 79. Despite that, few people have heard of it prior to being diagnosed with it, and it is not well understood at present.

For some time, it was thought that eating hard foods and the Western diet were the main contributing factors in the development of diverticular disease, but now scientists are less certain about the true causes of the disease.

There are still links drawn between constipation and diverticular disease, because it is certainly a problem with the functionality of the intestinal muscles, and increased strain seems a likely contributing factor for the issue. After all, if you overwork any part of your body, you can cause issues and wear it out more quickly. Prolonged pressure on your colon may have a negative impact. However, the exact cause of diverticular disease remains unknown, and the theory about intestinal pressure remains just that – a theory.

There is also minimal evidence to prove that a Western diet contributes, but it is certain that this disease is startlingly more common in Westernized societies, and there may be a link that has not yet been proven.

Whether a high-fiber diet helps to treat the problem caused by the disease or just reduce the number of flare-ups is also unclear, but it is certain that a high-fiber diet does help those who suffer. It reduces the pressure on the colon wall, and – unless you are experiencing diverticulitis – you should eat plenty of fiber to keep yourself healthier. Neglecting to do so can make episodes of pain and inflammation more common and possibly more severe.

You may decide to ignore information that say you should not eat corn, seeds, or nuts. There is little or no evidence about this, but for the convenience of readers who wish to avoid these foods, the recipes in this book won't include them. If you decide not to avoid them, you can easily add them to your meals.

Supplements to Help with Managing Diverticulitis Effectively

You should speak to your doctor before adding anything new to your diet, especially if you are currently suffering from any health problems, but there are a few additions that may help with diverticulitis and with preventing flare-ups. Discuss those that appeal to you with your health practitioner to see which may be suitable in your specific circumstances, or if they would advise against any.

Supplements

Unsurprisingly, the most useful thing you can take is often a fiber-supplement. These include methylcellulose or psyllium, both of which can help to reduce either constipation or diarrhea. Don't take them without reference to your doctor, however.

You should make sure that you drink some water at the same time as taking a fiber supplement, to ensure that you are getting enough liquid.

Digestive Enzymes

You may have heard about taking digestive enzymes. These are normally produced in the gut and they help to break down the food we eat. Few studies have been done on the usefulness of digestive enzymes, but some anecdotal evidence suggests that they may be able to ease certain stomach complaints.

Enzymes such as those found in pears and pineapples can reduce intestinal inflammation, so you may wish to either buy these enzymes (health food shops sometimes stock them) or make a point of including plenty of these fruits in your diet.

Drinks

What can you drink to help with diverticulitis? Well, there are a few options here. Some people believe that green tea helps to ease the symptoms of the disease, and it is thought to help fight infections, which may reduce your risk of a flare-up.

Ginger is also a popular option, so try some ginger tea if you are suffering from gastrointestinal complaints. This has been used for centuries for settling stomach aches, vomiting, and diarrhea.

Aloe vera is another popular option. It is thought to prevent constipation, which may reduce the risk of developing diverticular disease in the first place, and could reduce pain and stomach cramps. You shouldn't drink it in Large quantities, but two ounces a day may help to prevent symptoms.

Probiotics

Like the digestive enzymes, probiotics may give your digestive system the boost it needs to stay healthy. The term refers to the useful bacteria that reside in your gut and help aid digestion. Taking probiotics may reduce your risk of stomach issues.

Look for the Lactobacillus casei strain in particular, as these may be the most effective. You should be able to purchase powders or tablets, or you can eat live fermented foods, which should all contain probiotics.

A lot of people find that probiotics make their digestive system happier, and while this is again not a replacement for proper medical treatment, it is worth considering as a secondary approach to diverticular disease. Talk to your doctor before taking probiotics as research is still being done into their effectiveness, and there are no conclusive studies on it yet.

There is more information on gut microbes and diverticulitis in the following section.

Available Diverticulitis Treatments (Probiotics)

A person suffering from diverticulitis may be able to find some significant relief by taking probiotic supplements. In combination with other treatments the probiotic nutrients can give a person a whole new lease on life. There are some great food choices that already include probiotics in them. For example, eating foods with kefir, kimchi or kombucha in them will naturally help reduce the effects of diverticulitis.

Adding a supplement like Prescript Assist or VSL#3 is not a bad idea no matter where your health is currently at because it will improve your digestion and allow you to feel healthier each day.

Probiotics

It is important to make sure probiotics are in your diet. Probiotics will add healthy bacteria to the digestive system and make the colon work smoother and more efficiently which will allow for less development of Diverticular disease. Probiotics enhance the ability of the body to take the nutrients from food, break down lactose and even help improve the immune system of the body. Low fat yogurt or kefirs are a great source of probiotics for people to consume in order to avoid Diverticular disease.

Prebiotics are another option when it comes to correcting the level of good/bad bacteria in the digestive system. These are substances that are known to develop and nurture the growth and development of the positive forms of bacteria that will keep you healthy and manage your wellbeing.

This is exactly what a person is looking for when they need to restore a healthy bacterial balance. One great probiotic is fructose-oligosaccharide powder but consult a doctor or doctor to learn about more prebiotics that can help in solving a poor bacterial balance and help to stop diverticulitis before it begins.

Stay away for foods high in fat. It is no secret that foods that are high in fat tend to slow down the digestion process and can lead to episodes of constipation. This is not healthy for the colon because it causes undue stress on the muscles and can cause long term damage to them. It is also much easier to maintain a healthy weight if the foods that are high in fat are avoided.

Gut Microbiome and Diverticulitis

Bacteria and microorganisms are omnipresent: they live on the skin, in the nose, and the intestine. Our gastrointestinal system, particularly the Large intestine, is home to far more diverse populations. From the scientific point of view, doctors describe the complexity of microorganisms that live in humans with the term microbiota.

In recent times, medicine has shown much interest in life within the intestine; some have called it a "forgotten organ." A person's alimentary canal is the most densely populated ecosystem on Earth. About one hundred trillion microbes (bacteria, viruses, fungi) roam on the surface of the substantially oxygen-free intestine. It is a huge number, unimaginable. Written in numbers, it corresponds to 100,000,000,000,000 and is a thousand times greater than the number of stars that make up our galaxy.

If we put together all our intestinal microbes giving them the shape of an organ, this would weigh from 0.9 to 2.7 kg, compared to the brain weighing 1.2 kg. First, there was the talk of bacterial "flora" in the intestine. But this concept does not do justice to reality. The word flora is originated from the Latin, and it indicates the growth of plants on a portion of land, therefore something static.

Plants always remain in the same place. The concept of "bacterial flora" dates back to the period in which it was imagined that bacteria grew on the mucosa like grass on the earth and that the inside of the body was not touched. For this reason, we also talked about "bacterial carpet." Today we know that we are a dynamic whole and bacteria penetrate inside us, penetrating us.

They do not generate only in portions of the border. Everywhere, on and in our bodies, the surfaces, the passages between the inside and the outside are covered with biofilms of bacteria which in turn are formed by microbes that remain, comes and goes in a dynamic process. In the wake of the pioneering of the Human Genome Project, which has identified every human gene, scientists are now able to sequence Large amounts of DNA very quickly and cheaply.

Now it is even possible to identify dead microbes expelled from the body in defecation because their DNA remains intact. We felt that our microbes were not important, but science is beginning to reveal a different story to us. A story in which human life is intertwined with that of our hitchhikers, in which microbes manage the body, and it is not possible for the human body to be healthy without them.

How many genes are needed to form a human being? From the hypotheses of the group of the most prepared people on the planet surely a higher number, compared to the number of genes of the mice, which as we knew had 23,000.

With its timid 21,000 genes, the human genome is not much Larger than that of a worm. It is half that of the rice plant, and even the simple water flea with 31,000 genes outclasses it. Certainly, a complex and sophisticated body like the human body needs more proteins, and therefore more genes, than that of a worm.

But these 21,000 genes are not the only genes that govern our body. We do not live alone. Each of us is a superorganism. Our cells, although much Larger in weight and volume, are outnumbered in numbers, in the proportion of ten to one, by the cells of the microbes that live in and above us. Altogether, the microbes that live on the human body contain 4.4 million genes: here is the microbiome, the collective genome of the microbiota.

The Human Microbiome Project (HMP), a consortium of 200 researchers from 80 US research institutions in 5 years, analyzed the genome of microbes living on the human body, the microbiome, to identify which species are present.

From this variety of microorganisms, about 70% is in the gastrointestinal tract with a concentration that increases exponentially in the fecal-oral direction. All this population can be divided into two Large groups:
1. The autochthonous bacteria that start to colonize the digestive tract from birth and, after weaning, they turn into permanent, stable colonies. The quality and quantity of some particular strains can provide such constant "imprinting" that it can be used for individual identification with a precision higher than that of fingerprints!
2. The allochthones bacteria is found in our intestine only in a short form without forming stable colonies, and they are introduced with food when their number increases they cause imbalances that from simple dysbiosis can reach even more serious diseases.

   As we proceed inside the gastrointestinal system, the environmental conditions change, and this determines the variety of microbial species that settle at different levels. The bacteria colonize the segments of the intestinal tube where they find the most suitable conditions for their development: however, anatomy and physiology are essential in determining the quantity and quality of microorganisms. In general, traits, where the contractile movement of the intestine (peristalsis) is more contained, are welcome.

Among the factors that regulate the balance of the bacterial population is the pH, which is the acidity or basicity of the environment, oxygen, nutrients, and the presence of competitors. All the bacteria that live in the gastrointestinal tract are also found in the faeces whose composition reproduces the balance that has been established in recent stretches.
In inflammatory bowel diseases, and not only, instead of a functioning microbiome, there is also a disorder in the intestinal microbes, and the result is an excess or defect of metabolic products, genetic activations, and enzymes.

This condition is called "dysbiosis." The term originated from the Greek words dys for "wrong," "disturbed" and bios for "life" and the ending "-osi" for "condition," "state." A simple way to identify a dysbiosis is the control of the stool surfacing in the toilet (correct eubiosis) compared to a sinking (dysbiosis in progress).

Why Do Our Bodies Need Bacteria?

The intestinal bacteria produce substances that act on the brain through the intestinal mucosa and cover different ways: blood, immune, and nervous. They carry out an enormous metabolic job and constitute a precious ecosystem that, if intact, is very important for health and well-being.

"The microbiota can be seen as a metabolic" organ "tuned to our physiology." (Backhed, 2004) They play a vital role in the digestion, assimilation, and elimination of food. Without bacteria it would be impossible to digest certain types of fiber properly. They feed and digest them for us, and in doing so, they also produce some nutrients we need.

Depending on the diet, the bacteria release a particular amount of active metabolic substances. The vitamins belong to these. Certain Bifidus and Escherichia Coli strains produce, as it was discovered in 1983, vitamins of the B group: B1, B2, B3 and their nicotinamide derivatives, B5, B6, B12, folic acid, biotin and vitamin K necessary for blood coagulation.

For their metabolism, for example, nerve cells need vitamin B12 and folic acid, both of which are supplied by food through the action of intestinal bacteria. Even a minimal deficiency of these trace elements can cause an insufficient supply to the nerves which have repercussions in the form of nervous weakness in the belly-brain-belly agreement.

The intestinal bacteria also perform a detoxifying function, neutralizing, for example, some substances that are harmful to our body, such as ammonia. The unhealthy microbiota developed, increases the levels of pro-inflammatory cytokines, such as IL-6 and IL-8 and lipopolysaccharide (LPS), which cause intestinal inflammation and permeability of the walls.

Furthermore, these inflammatory molecules contribute to the metabolic dysfunction with the altered metabolism of bile acid, the production of short-chain fatty acids, the secretion of the intestinal hormone, and the circulation of branched-chain amino acids. The most important role bacteria play in the reabsorption of bile acids. Bile is composed of bile salts, the bilirubin dye, cholesterol, and phospholipids. These are important for bile stabilization.

If the bile is salty, bilirubin or cholesterol crystallize, gallstones form, based on their relationship with phospholipids. Bile is formed in liver cells and the gall bladder and from there, depending on food intake, released into the Small intestine. Bile also contains several enzymes and substances that the liver has Filtered to purify the body.

If the intestine is not healthy, it can leave the liver with a more significant number of toxic substances through the bile to detoxify, then brought back into the intestine, through which they should be eliminated. If the microbiome is in good shape here, the intestinal bacteria carry out the steps necessary for detoxification; otherwise, they may be reabsorbed and returned to the liver.

Great attention was paid to the possible role of short chain fatty acids (SCFA acronym for Short Chain Fatty Acids) such as butyrate, propionate, and acetate since SCFA are the main product of the digestive action of intestinal microbiota. It has been reported that SCFAs affect host metabolism through various parallel pathways associated with protein-coupled receptors, and these receptors are active in neuroendocrine cells in the intestine and can, therefore, influence brain signaling.

The more a disturbance persists in the intestinal mucosa, in the form of a reduction in the number of microbes, a modified composition, a lack of mucosa, inflammation, immune reactions and the higher the probability that the cells of the intestinal epithelium do what they want.

For nerve cells to at least be able to transmit impulses to other cells, communication, a compatible instrument is necessary for everyone. These are nerve messengers, neurotransmitters. Small molecules that are transported by a nerve cell in the space of the next one. Serotonin is one of the most vital neurotransmitters, and it is found mainly in the intestine. Its effects on the body affect all central, and vital areas: like the heart and circulation of blood coagulation, or regulation of eye pressure. It transmits mucosal stimuli to the tissues in the gastrointestinal tract, and as a result of this, the movements of the organs are coordinated.

Also, it occurs directly or indirectly, in almost all the functions of the central nervous system and of the enteric ones: the serotonin rule perception, sensitivity and temperature, tiredness and pain, stimulus development, hormonal production, and sexual behavior.

If there is enough serotonin in the body, the human being is balanced, if the serotonin is lacking, moods appear as prostration and killing, up to depression, dissatisfaction, irritability, fear, and aggressive behavior. It also performs protective functions and increases the barrier effect: increased production of mucin and zoludin is a component of the tight junctions (the tight junctions that allow the intestinal epithelium to act as a protective barrier towards the inside of the body).

Finally, the intestinal microbiota is essential for our immune system. About 70-80% of the body's immune cells are located in the intestine. The microbiota stimulates the maturation of the immune system and has a "barrier effect" against potential aggressors. The "good" bacteria (saprophytes or commensals) attach themselves to the intestinal wall and occupy the space, thus preventing the establishment of harmful bacteria.

Bacteria make the nerves grow or prevent its growth, and they make the connections grow or prevent them, inhibit, favor, or regulate. Bacteria determine brain activity, the values of blood and tissues of neurotransmitters, hormones, and hematocytes, as well as development and inflammation and vegetative reactions, depend on them. Intestinal bacteria is the part that accompanies us throughout our lives, and the brain development of our ability to feel, to behave and even to think, without them, we will not be a whole human being.

Some microorganisms can produce a neurotransmitter, gamma-aminobutyric acid. This substance, abbreviated as GABA, is one of the most abundant signaling molecules in the nervous system, which keeps the emotional part of our brain, the limbic system, under control. But it would be possible to use this knowledge to treat anxiety disorders with GABA-producing microbes in the form of probiotics.

So how does this all tie in with Diverticulitis?

When diverticulitis, like other digestive illnesses are caused by excessive proliferation of harmful bacteria or poor differentiation of bacterial strains, the microbiota will produce harmful effects on the rest of the body and then to the brain. The "bad" bacteria will produce toxic substances, called "neurotoxins," for the nervous system.

These neurotoxins will eventually alter mental functions, generating stress, anxiety, and even psychiatric or neurodegenerative diseases. An imbalance in the intestinal microbiota will have the effect of depleting or over-stimulating the immune system. The harmful bacteria that prevail over those beneficial alters of the intestinal wall can make it porous, allowing the passage of macromolecules and foreign toxins into the blood.

These intruders cause the immediate reaction of intestinal immune cells, which will alert the entire immune system, releasing inflammatory molecules and stress hormones. In this way, the harmful intestinal bacteria can start a state of chronic inflammation, with negative effects on the brain and our mental health.

How to Prevent Attacks

You may not always be able to prevent an attack of diverticulitis, but it is important to try and minimize them, mostly for the sake of your comfort and well-being. An attack can leave you in a lot of pain, and will often result in the need for rest, possibly coupled with antibiotics and a clear liquid diet.

It is not known exactly what causes attacks of diverticulitis, but if you drop too much fiber from your diet, you may find that you have problems. It is a good idea to keep a record of how much fiber you are consuming most days. If you notice that your stools have become hard or uncomfortable, take action quickly to resolve this.

Fiber pulls more water into stools, making them softer, and putting less pressure on your digestive system as a result. Remember to include a variety of fibrous foods, such as fruits and vegetables, as well as whole grains.

Of course, fiber can't pull in water if there isn't enough water in your system, so being hydrated is important too. You may be able to reduce the risk of attacks by drinking plenty of water and exercising well. Exercise helps to tone your intestinal muscles, strengthening them and making them more resistant to diverticulitis. It also encourages more frequent and comfortable bowel movements, which reduces the pressure on your digestive system.

No specific foods are known to cause diverticulitis, so there isn't anything you should particularly avoid. In general, diets that are high in red meat and sugar are thought to be less healthy, so it is a good idea to reduce these to boost your overall health, but there isn't a known connection between them and flare-ups. Indeed, it has proven very hard for doctors to pinpoint what does cause issues.

When you aren't suffering from a flare-up, you may wish to try avoiding white bread, white rice, and white pasta, as these are low in fiber and contribute to constipation. The wholegrain alternatives are considered a better option for diverticulitis prevention, and should help to reduce the risk of attacks.

If you do choose to take laxatives to make movements easier, discuss this with your doctor, as long-term use could cause other issues.

You may not be able to completely prevent diverticulitis, but you can lower the risk of attacks and make your system work more smoothly by being careful about your diet. You may also improve your overall health in this way.

How to Calm Down a Diverticulitis Episode

If you are suffering from an attack, you should first discuss the problems with your doctor. The advice will differ depending on your personal circumstances and the severity of the problem. Always refer to a professional before deciding how to treat an episode, as you might make a problem worse if you take the wrong approach to it.

It is also possible that you will need antibiotics, so talking to your doctor is important. They will be able to assess how bad the episode is and what treatment is required. If you are given antibiotics, don't stop taking them before you have completed the full course, even if your symptoms improve.

If your doctor advises you to swap to a clear liquid diet, make sure you do so, and follow up with them about how it's working and when to come off it. You should aim to get back onto solid food as soon as you are able to, so work with your healthcare practitioner to make sure this happens. It isn't fun or healthy to be on a liquid diet for longer than necessary.

However, common advice is to take it very easy on your digestive system. Whether or not your doctor would recommend you move onto a clear liquid diet, you might find that you feel better more quickly if you reduce the amount of fiber in your diet for a while. Try white bread and pasta, and eat a little less than you usually would (if you are still eating, of course).

You may find that applying a heat pad or hot water bottle to your abdomen helps to ease the pain a bit. Don't go for extreme heat, but gentle warmth, and hold it or lean it against your abdomen for as long as feels good to you. A hot bath may also reduce your symptoms and make you more comfortable, although you should again aim for comfortable rather than extreme heat.

Try to relax, too. This can be very difficult if you're in pain, and knowing that you should do so often creates a vicious cycle of increasing pain, so look into meditation and deep breathing techniques. While these can be difficult to apply when the pain is intense, they will help overall, and are well worth learning. There are many online resources that will assist you with this.

Finally, you may find that non-prescription painkillers help too. Tylenol is commonly advised as being effective. You should keep some in to help you deal with flare-ups.

When you start feeling better, begin slowly increasing the amount of fiber in your diet. Remember to drink plenty of water as you do this, because this prevents constipation and will also help you to feel better.

You should take it easy while you are feeling ill, and don't do anything too strenuous. Resting will allow your body to focus on healing the inflammation. You can do some gentle exercises and stretching if you feel up to it, but you should allow your body time to heal, rather than encouraging it to do more work.

Approved Diverticulitis Foods

It is important to remember that having diverticulitis does not mean that there are going to be any symptoms visible for a person to observe. Many live blissfully unaware of their condition until they have an attack and then that painful uncomfortable situation will need to be treated by a medical professional. One of the simple cures is with antibiotics but there are more serious cases that need to be handled with surgery.

Again, we know that if you are suffering from diverticulitis, a liquid diet may be prescribed by your doctor as being included in your treatment. This will give the colon a chance to heal and recover without having to perform the task that it was designed for.

This type of liquid diet should include tea, water, ice pops, broth and fruit juices. Very slowly the patient can start to readd solid foods back in your diet. However, they really need to stop neglecting the fiber at this point and start to eat high fiber foods. Because of the medical condition the colon might have difficulty at first passing high fiber foods very well so your doctor will most likely prescribe foods that are lower in fiber to begin with.

These include eggs, fish, poultry and all dairy products as well. Remember the more fiber that is present in the diet the more bulk there will be in the stool and that will reduce the pressure on the colon to perform its job.

There have been studies done that demonstrate quite clearly that foods that are rich in fiber helps to curve the onset of diverticulitis and the flares it brings to the table. Again, it is urged that you be sure to consume at least 25 grams of fiber daily.

Phases/Stages of the Diverticulitis Diet & How To Eat During Each Phase

There are three main phases of the Diverticulitis diet: eating during an active flare-up, eating while recovering from a flare, and preventing a flare in the future. As with any other diet, you will need to listen to your body throughout each stage and adjust the diet slowly as you add new foods while closely monitoring your symptoms.

Phase 1: Clear Fluids (During A Flare)

While going through an active flare, your symptoms can become extreme. Due to this it's smart for you to give your bowel a period of rest. As you can imagine the best way to do this is by sticking to a clear fluid diet. This will aid in your recovery as your body may outright reject solid foods.

It is vital to note that the clear fluid stage of the diet is NOT intended to be a long-term diet. In fact, the general expectation is that you remain in this stage for no more than a couple of days.

Please Note:
Restricting yourself to a clear fluid diet for an excessive amount of time may cause you to feel light-headed, weak, hungry, and fatigued. You can also experience muscle wasting, excessive weight loss, and depletion of vitamins and minerals.

This occurs due to the fact that it's incredibly difficult to meet the body's daily caloric requirements for fat, protein, and carbohydrates through a clear fluid diet. The average person will need to provide their body with at least 200 grams of carbohydrates to have enough energy to go through the day. If you struggle with low blood sugar, diabetes, or other blood sugar challenges, you may want to monitor your blood sugar levels during this stage.

As the name implies, this phase is composed of clear liquids. These include green tea, Fresh fruit juice, clear broth, and gelatin dessert. The clear liquid diet provides the body with salt, liquids, and enough nutrients to function temporarily, **generally for a few days,** until you can eat normal food.

Phase 2: Low-Residue/Low Fiber Diet (Immediately After A Controlled Flare)

A low-residue (or low-fiber) diet acts as the reintroduction phase, after your flare-up symptoms have mostly passed but before your body is ready for high-fiber or high residue foods.

Phase 3: High Fiber Meals (Daily Life/ Preventing Future Flares)

This final stage in the diverticulitis diet is the High Fiber diet. This stage is used to maintain a balanced diet while preventing a future flare. It is basically your general day to day eating routine, and generally takes up the majority of your diverticulitis eating plan.

It is important to note, however, that you do not want to jump directly from a significantly low fiber diet (such as a clear fluid diet) directly to a high fiber diet, as this will do more harm to your colon than good. It is always best to ease into any stage of the plan that requires an increase in your fiber intake.

Aim to increase your fiber intake by 2 to 4 grams per week until you reach the recommended amount for your age and biology. Bear in mind that as you increase your fiber, you also need to increase your water intake to help move the fiber through your intestinal tract.

Essential Shopping List

Fruits
- [ ] Apple Sauce
- [ ] Apples
- [ ] Apricots
- [ ] Bananas
- [ ] Dates
- [ ] Mangoes
- [ ] Oranges
- [ ] Peaches
- [ ] Prunes

Juices
- [ ] Apple Juice
- [ ] Lemon Juice
- [ ] Lime Juice
- [ ] Orange Juice
- [ ] Cranberry Juice

Vegetables
- [ ] Alfalfa Sprouts
- [ ] Artichoke Hearts
- [ ] Asparagus
- [ ] Avocados
- [ ] Black Olives
- [ ] Broccoli
- [ ] Butternut Squash
- [ ] Cabbage
- [ ] Carrots
- [ ] Cauliflower
- [ ] Celery
- [ ] Eggplants
- [ ] Garlic
- [ ] Green Bell peppers (seedless)
- [ ] Green Olives
- [ ] Scallions
- [ ] Leeks
- [ ] Mushrooms
- [ ] Lettuce
- [ ] Olives
- [ ] Onions
- [ ] Peas (frozen, cooked)
- [ ] Pimento
- [ ] Red bell peppers (seedless)
- [ ] Russet Potatoes
- [ ] Shallots
- [ ] Spinach
- [ ] Sugar Snap Peas
- [ ] Summer Squash
- [ ] Yellow Peppers (seedless)
- [ ] Tomatoes (seedless)
- [ ] Water chestnuts
- [ ] Zucchini
- [ ] Sweet Yams

Beans & Peas
- [ ] Black Beans
- [ ] Butter Beans
- [ ] Cannellini Beans
- [ ] Garbanzo Beans
- [ ] Canned Kidney Beans
- [ ] Lentils
- [ ] Canned Lima Beans
- [ ] Canned Navy Beans
- [ ] Canned Red Beans

Grains, Breads & Other Starches
- [ ] All Bran Cereal
- [ ] Barley
- [ ] Brown Rice
- [ ] Fiber One Cereal
- [ ] Long Grain Rice
- [ ] Oat Bran
- [ ] Rolled Oats
- [ ] Whole Wheat Tortellini
- [ ] Whole Wheat Flour
- [ ] Whole Wheat Pasta
- [ ] Whole Wheat Pita

- ☐ Whole Wheat Tortillas
- ☐ Whole Wheat Bread

Meats
- ☐ Crab Meat, Cooked
- ☐ Ground Chicken, Lean
- ☐ Ground Turkey, Lean
- ☐ Lean Ham
- ☐ Shrimp, Large, peeled
- ☐ Canned Tuna Fish, in water
- ☐ Turkey Breast
- ☐ Chicken Breast

Dairy
- ☐ Cheddar Cheese (low fat)
- ☐ Cottage Cheese (low fat)
- ☐ Cream Cheese (low fat)
- ☐ Feta Cheese
- ☐ Monterrey Jack Cheese (low fat)
- ☐ Parmesan Cheese
- ☐ Eggs
- ☐ Half and half cream
- ☐ Milk, low fat
- ☐ Yogurt, low fat

Spices, Herbs & Oils
- ☐ Baking Powder
- ☐ Basil (Fresh or dried)
- ☐ Canola Oil
- ☐ Cilantro (Fresh)

- ☐ Cinnamon powder
- ☐ Cumin
- ☐ Curry Powder
- ☐ Dill, (Fresh or dried)
- ☐ Italian Seasoning
- ☐ Nutmeg
- ☐ Olive Oil
- ☐ Oregano, (Fresh and dried)
- ☐ Parsley, Italian (Fresh)
- ☐ Sage (Fresh)
- ☐ Tarragon (Fresh)
- ☐ Thyme (Fresh and dried)
- ☐ Vanilla

Condiments
- ☐ Vegetable Stock
- ☐ Chicken Stock
- ☐ Coconut Milk
- ☐ Dijon Mustard
- ☐ Honey
- ☐ Light Ranch Dressing
- ☐ Maple Syrup
- ☐ Tomato Paste
- ☐ Tomato Sauce
- ☐ Tomato Puree
- ☐ Canned Tomato, diced, seedless
- ☐
- ☐ Mayonnaise, low fat
- ☐ Red Wine Vinegar
- ☐ Rice Vinegar
- ☐ Soy Sauce
- ☐ Sweet Pickle Relish
- ☐ Tarragon Vinegar

List of Foods to Avoid

Patients with diverticulitis are often urged to exercise caution when consuming seeds or anything with seeds (i.e., tomatoes, melons, berries, etc.). Small foods particles such as seeds are theorized to potentially be able to get logged in the diverticulum and cause inflammation.

Although there hasn't been any scientific evidence to date that would confirm this belief, you may prefer to stick with the previous advice. I will be including seeds and nuts in our Foods to Avoid list and omit them from my recipes.

Be sure to consult your doctor to see whether you would be permitted to including them in your diet.

There are several reasons why certain foods should be avoided during the acute (symptomatic) phase of diverticulitis. Some of these reasons include:

- Increase the bulk of the stool: Some of these foods are high in fiber and, therefore, contribute to the consistency and bulk of the stool. In many cases, as a person already suffers from severe constipation, increased intake of such foods will only make it harder to defecate and will eventually result in more abdominal discomfort.

- Some of these foods can get caught in the pouches called diverticula.

- Take longer time for digestion: Some of these foods take a longer time to digest. As the digestive system is already sore (inflamed), and under abnormally high-pressure during diverticulitis, more of such foods will only create more complications, and as a result, the stomach and intestines would not get the "rest" they need the most during diverticulitis.

- Produce flatulence and bloating: Intestinal gas and bloating are common side effects of a high fiber diet. Presence of such symptoms will increase the risk of more complications in diverticulitis attack.

Vegetables with Small Particles or Seeds
- Cucumber (only English is acceptable)
- Green Peppers (Acceptable if seeds are removed)
- Tomato (Acceptable if seeds are removed)
- Chili Peppers
- Corn

Seeds & Nuts
- Avoid all types

Sweets with Small Particles or Seeds
- Nutty Candy
- Fruit Jam with Seeds
- Nutty Desserts
- Raisins with Seeds

Fruits with Small Particles or Seeds
- Blackberries
- Blueberries
- Coconut (dried)
- Whole Cranberries (Cranberry Relish)
- Figs
- Grapes with seeds
- Kiwi
- Pomegranates
- Raspberries
- Strawberries
- Watermelon (Acceptable if seedless)

Starches (Refined)
- Bread or rolls with nuts/seeds
- Popcorn
- Wild Rice

Diverticulitis FAQ

What is the significance of the Diverticulitis Diet?

While a typical diverticulitis diet itself, is not considered a sole treatment for diverticulitis, it does strengthen the overall effect of the therapy, and ensures rapid healing and fast improvement in symptoms. In other words, a diverticulitis diet helps people while they are still on the treatment and ensures better healing rates and improvement in symptoms. A diverticulitis diet also eases the burden from the digestive during the diverticulitis treatment.

What is a clear fluid diet?

As the name implies, this diet is composed of clear liquids and foods that are liquid at room temperature. These include green tea, Fresh fruit juice, clear broth, and gelatin dessert. The clear liquid diet provides the body with salt, liquids, and enough nutrients to function temporarily, **generally for a few days,** until you can eat normal food.

What are the side effects or risks involved with a Clear Fluid Diet?

As stated throughout the previous chapters, the clear fluid s does not have a sufficient amount of nutrients, one should not take a clear liquid diet for more than 2-3 days, unless your dietician or the doctor has asked you to do so.

Always remember to consult your nutritionist, doctor, or health care provider for any queries you may have about your clear fluid diet plan.
Your doctor or health care provider will also tell you how much fluid you may have on daily basis.

Important NOTE: a clear fluid diet is not a "well-balanced" diet and is not recommended for otherwise normal individuals

When to use the diverticulitis diet?

During "uncomplicated" diverticulosis: An uncomplicated diverticulosis simply means the presence of diverticula in the Large intestine (colon), before the stage of inflammation or diverticulitis occurs. Therefore, before the development of "diverticulitis" stage, the recommended diet will be a high fiber diet.

When a patient suffers from severe symptoms, such as lower abdominal pain, fever, vomiting, and constipation, and is considered to be experiencing a flare, the diverticulitis diet is implemented. The recommended diet for this phase is clear liquids and a low-fiber diet to follow (explained in detail in previous chapters).

Who gets Diverticulosis and Diverticular infection?

Diverticulosis turns out to be more normal as individual's age, especially in individuals more established than age 50.3 Some individuals with Diverticulosis create diverticulitis, and the quantity of cases is expanding.

In spite of the fact that Diverticular disease is for the most part thought to be a condition found in more seasoned grown-ups, it is turning out to be more regular in individuals more youthful than age 50, the greater part of whom are male.

When would a Clear Fluid diet be needed?

A clear fluid diet is indicated in the following conditions:

When you cannot properly digest (break down) solid foods e.g. dehydration, vomiting, diarrhea, after surgery of intestines, or in certain chronic diseases.

When experiencing a diverticulitis flare, a clear liquid diet is advised.

Symptomatic improvement usually occurs within 2-3 days, at which point patients are recommended to slowly reintroduce fiber to their diet.

What is the benefit, if any, of a clear fluid diet?

The basic benefit of a clear liquid diet is that it helps one feel better until he or she is able to eat solid food.

What is the recommended dose of fiber and water per day?

The recommended intake of fiber is generally:

    Women age 19 to 50 = 25 grams per day

    Women age 50+ = 21 grams per day

    Men age 19 to 50 = 38 grams per day

    Men age 50+ = 30 grams per day

While the recommended water intake is generally:

    Men age 19+ = 12 cups (about 3 liters) per day

    Women age 19+ = 9 cups (about 2 liters) per day

Please contact your doctor to confirm that these values are okay for your specific scenario.

Are there any side effects?

Naturally, as a clear liquid diet lacks solid or semi solid food, you may have diarrhea (loose, watery stools), nausea and vomiting (throwing up), and flatulence when you are on this kind of diet.

What is fiber?

Fiber is a substance in foods that originates from plants. Fiber diminishes stool so it moves easily through the colon and is less demanding to pass. Solvent fiber disintegrates in water and is found in beans, organic product, and oat items.

Insoluble fiber does not break down in water and is found in entire grain items and vegetables. Both sorts of fiber forestall stoppage. Obstruction is a condition in which a grown-up has less than three solid discharges a week or has defecations with stools that are hard, dry, and little, making them excruciating or hard to pass.

High-fiber foods likewise have numerous advantages in counteracting and controlling incessant maladies, for example, cardiovascular illness, stoutness, diabetes, and disease.

What are the symptoms of a Diverticular Infection?

Individuals with diverticulitis may have numerous symptoms, the most widely recognized of which agony in the lower is left half of the stomach area. The torment is normally serious and goes ahead all of a sudden; however, it can likewise be gentle and afterward decline more than a few days. The force of the agony can vacillate.

Consult With Your Doctor

Whenever you are in doubt or have questions about diverticular disease and your experience of it, talk to your doctor. While you will probably soon learn tips and tricks that make you feel better, and you may be able to manage your condition well through a careful diet, you should be in regular contact with your GP and keep them up to date on how you're feeling and any flare-ups you experience.

They will be able to offer advice on the symptoms, the episodes, and the general care needed to handle this disease. Ask questions or pass information on to them regularly so they can stay up to date about how you're feeling, and take prompt action if something is required.

While you may find that diverticulitis is not such a problem for you if your diet is good, you should still consult with your doctor from time to time, even if all you do is let them know that you're feeling well and not having any problems. Good communication is key to handling any condition, and diverticular disease is no exception to that rule.

Phase: 1- Clear Liquid Recipes

Orange Juice

Servings|2 Time|10 minutes
Nutritional Content (per serving)
Cal| 346   Fat| 0.9g   Protein| 6.9g   Carbs| 86.5g   Fiber| 17.7g

Ingredients:
- ❖ Oranges (8, peeled and sectioned)

Directions:
1. Add the orange sections into a juicer and extract the juice according to the manufacturer's method.
2. Through a cheesecloth-lined strainer, strain the juice and transfer into 2 glasses.
3. Serve immediately.

Apple Juice

Servings|2 Time|10 minutes
Nutritional Content (per serving):
Cal| 464   Fat| 1.6g   Protein| 2.4g   Carbs| 122.6g   Fiber| 21.6g

Ingredients:
- ❖ Medium apples (8, cored and quartered)

Directions:
1. Add the apples into a juicer and extract the juice according to the manufacturer's method.
2. Through a cheesecloth-lined strainer, strain the juice and transfer into 2 glasses.
3. Serve immediately.

Citrus Apple Juice

Servings|2 Time|10 minutes
Nutritional Content (per serving):
Cal| 348   Fat| 1.3g   Protein| 2.4g   Carbs| 90.6g   Fiber| 14g

Ingredients:
- Large apples (5, cored and chopped)
- Small lemon (1)
- Fresh orange juice (1 cup)

Directions:
1. Place all the ingredients in a blender and pulse until well combined.
2. Through a cheesecloth-lined strainer, strain the juice and transfer into 2 glasses.
3. Serve immediately.

Grapes Juice

Servings|3 Time|10 minutes
Nutritional Content (per serving):
Cal| 41   Fat| 0.2g   Protein| 0.4g   Carbs| 10.5g   Fiber| 10g

Ingredients:
- White seedless grapes (2 cups)
- Ice cubes (6-8)
- Filtered water (1½ cups)

Directions:
1. Place all the ingredients in a blender and pulse until well combined.
2. Through a cheesecloth-lined strainer, strain the juice and transfer into 3 glasses.
3. Serve immediately.

Lemony Grapes Juice

Servings|3   Time|10 minutes
Nutritional Content (per serving)
Cal| 85   Fat| 0.5g   Protein| 0.9g   Carbs| 21.3g   Fiber| 1.1g

Ingredients:
- ❖ Seedless white grapes (4 cups)
- ❖ Fresh lemon juice (2 tablespoons)

Directions:
1. Place all the ingredients in a blender and pulse until well combined.
2. Through a cheesecloth-lined strainer, strain the juice and transfer into 3 glasses.
3. Serve immediately.

Grapes & Apple Juice

Servings|2   Time|10 minutes
Nutritional Content (per serving):
Cal| 352   Fat| 1.3g   Protein| 2.1g   Carbs| 29.8g   Fiber| 14.3g

Ingredients:
- ❖ Large green apples (5, cored and sliced)
- ❖ Seedless white grapes (2 cups)
- ❖ Fresh lime juice (2 teaspoons)

Directions:
1. Add all ingredients into a juicer and extract the juice according to the manufacturer's method.
2. Through a cheesecloth-lined strainer, strain the juice and transfer into 2 glasses.
3. Serve immediately.

Strawberry Juice

Servings|2 . Time|10 minutes
Nutritional Content (per serving):
Cal| 49   Fat| 0.5g   Protein| 1g   Carbs| 11.6g   Fiber| 3g

Ingredients:
- ❖ Fresh strawberries (2½ cups, hulled)
- ❖ Fresh lime juice (1 teaspoon)
- ❖ Filtered water (2 cups)

Directions:
1. Place all the ingredients in a blender and pulse until well combined.
2. Through a cheesecloth-lined strainer, strain the juice and transfer into 3 glasses.
3. Serve immediately.

Cranberry Juice

Servings|4   Time|10 minutes
Nutritional Content (per serving):
Cal| 66   Fat| 0g   Protein| 0g   Carbs| 11.5g   Fiber| 4g

Ingredients:
- ❖ Fresh cranberries (4 cups)
- ❖ Filtered water (2 cups)
- ❖ Fresh lemon juice (1 tablespoon)
- ❖ Raw honey (1 teaspoon)

Directions:
1. Place all the ingredients in a blender and pulse until well combined.
2. Through a cheesecloth-lined strainer, strain the juice and transfer into 4 glasses.
3. Serve immediately.

Carrot & Orange Juice

Servings|4   Time|10 minutes
Nutritional Content (per serving):
Cal| 183   Fat| 0.2g   Protein| 3.7g   Carbs| 44.8g   Fiber| 10.2g

Ingredients:
- ❖ Carrots (2 pounds, trimmed and scrubbed)
- ❖ Small oranges (6, peeled and sectioned)

Directions:
1. Add the carrots and orange sections into a juicer and extract the juice according to the manufacturer's method.
2. Through a cheesecloth-lined strainer, strain the juice and transfer into 4 glasses.
3. Serve immediately.

Mixed Fruit Punch

Servings|12   Time|15 minutes
Nutritional Content (per serving):
Cal| 97   Fat| 0.3g   Protein| 1.3g   Carbs| 23.3g   Fiber| 1.7g

Ingredients:
- ❖ Fresh pineapple juice (3 cups)
- ❖ Fresh orange juice (2 cups)
- ❖ seedless watermelon (2 cups, cut into bite-sized chunks)
- ❖ Oranges (2, peeled and cut into wedges)
- ❖ Diet lemon lime soda (24-fluid ounces canned)
- ❖ Fresh ruby red grapefruit juice (1 cup)
- ❖ Fresh lime juice (¼ cup)
- ❖ Fresh pineapple (2 cups, cut into bite-sized chunks)
- ❖ Limes (2, quartered)
- ❖ Lemon (1, sliced)
- ❖ Crushed ice, as required

Directions:
1. In a large pitcher, add all ingredients except for soda cans and ice and stir to combine. Set aside for 30 minutes.
2. Through a cheesecloth-lined strainer, strain the punch into another large pitcher.
3. Fill the glasses with ice and top with punch about ¾ of the way.
4. Pour in the soda and serve.

Lemonade

Servings|4   Time|10 minutes
Nutritional Content (per serving)
Cal| 4   Fat| 0.1g   Protein| 0.1g   Carbs| 0.3g   Fiber| 0.1g

Ingredients:
- ❖ Filtered water (4½ cups)
- ❖ Stevia extract (3-4 drops)
- ❖ Fresh lemon juice (¼ cup)
- ❖ Ice cubes, as required

Directions:
1. In a pitcher, place the water, lemon juice and stevia and mix well.
2. Through a cheesecloth-lined strainer, strain the lemonade in another pitcher.
3. Refrigerate for 30-40 minutes.
4. Add ice cubes in serving glasses and fill with lemonade.
5. Serve chilled.

Apple & Lime Sports Drink

Servings|4   Time|10 minutes
Nutritional Content (per serving):
Cal| 30   Fat| 0g   Protein| 0.1g   Carbs| 7.8g   Fiber| 0.1g

Ingredients:
- ❖ Spring water (3½ cups)
- ❖ Fresh lime juice (1 teaspoon)
- ❖ Sea salt (¼ teaspoon)
- ❖ Fresh apple juice (2 cups)
- ❖ Honey (1 tablespoon)

Directions:
1. In a large pitcher, add all ingredients and stir to combine.
2. Through a cheesecloth-lined strainer, strain the punch into another large pitcher.
3. Refrigerate to chill before serving.

Orange, Lemon & Lime Sports Drink

Servings|4 Time|10 minutes
Nutritional Content (per serving):
Cal| 36   Fat| 0.1g   Protein| 0.2g   Carbs| 8.9g   Fiber| 0.1g

Ingredients:

- ❖ Cold water (4½ cups, divided)
- ❖ Fresh lime juice (2 tablespoons)
- ❖ Salt (¼ teaspoon)
- ❖ Fresh orange juice (1/3 cup)
- ❖ Fresh lemon juice (2 tablespoons)
- ❖ Honey (1½ tablespoons)

Directions:
1. In a large pitcher, add all ingredients and stir to combine.
2. Through a cheesecloth-lined strainer, strain the punch into another large pitcher.
3. Refrigerate to chill before serving.

Chilled Green Tea

Servings|6 Time|13 minutes
Nutritional Content (per serving):
Cal| 46   Fat| 0.1g   Protein| 0.1g   Carbs| 12.2g   Fiber| 0.2g

Ingredients:

- ❖ Filtered water (5 cups)
- ❖ Fresh lemon juice (¼ cup, strained)
- ❖ Honey (¼ cup)
- ❖ Green tea bags (5)
- ❖ Fresh lime juice (¼ cup, strained)
- ❖ Ice cubes, as required

Directions:
1. In a medium pan, add 2 cups of water and bring to a boil.
2. Add in the tea bags and turn off the heat.
3. Immediately, cover the pan and steep for 3-4 minutes.
4. With a large spoon, gently press the tea bags against the pan to extract the tea completely.
5. Remove the tea bags from the pan and discard them.
6. Add honey and stir until dissolved.
7. In a large pitcher, place the tea, lemon and lime juice and stir to combine.
8. Add remaining cold water and stir to combine.
9. Refrigerate to chill before serving.
10. Add ice cubes in serving glasses and fill with tea.

Citrus Green Tea

Servings|4 Time|14 minutes
Nutritional Content (per serving):
Cal| 11   Fat| 0g   Protein| 0g   Carbs| 3g   Fiber| 0.1g

Ingredients:
- ❖ Filtered water (4½ cups)
- ❖ Lemon peel strips (4)
- ❖ Honey (1½ tablespoons)
- ❖ Orange peel strips (4)
- ❖ Green tea bags (4)

Directions:
1. In a medium pan, add the water, orange and lemon peel strips over medium-high heat and bring to a boil.
2. Now adjust the heat to low and simmer, uncovered, for about 10 minutes.
3. With a slotted spoon, remove the orange and lemon peel strips and discard them.
4. Add in the tea bags and turn off the heat.
5. Immediately, cover the pan and steep for 3 minutes.
6. With a large spoon, gently press the tea bags against the pan to extract the tea completely.
7. Remove the tea bags from the pan and discard them.
8. Add honey and stir until dissolved.
9. Strain the tea in mugs and serve immediately.

Simple Black Tea

Servings|2 Time|13 minutes

Nutritional Content (per serving):

Cal| 11   Fat| 0g   Protein| 0g   Carbs| 2.9g   Fiber| 0g

Ingredients:
- ❖ Filtered water (2 cups)
- ❖ Honey (1 teaspoon)
- ❖ Black tea leaves (½ teaspoon)

Directions:
1. In a pan, add the water and bring to a boil.
2. Stir in the tea leaves and turn off the heat.
3. Immediately, cover the pan and steep for 3 minutes.
4. Add honey and stir until dissolved.
5. Strain the tea in mugs and serve immediately.

Lemony Black Tea

Servings|6 Time|10 minutes
Nutritional Content (per serving)
Cal| 1 Fat| 0g Protein| 0g Carbs| 0.2g Fiber| 0g

Ingredients:
- ❖ Black tea leaves (tablespoon)
- ❖ Cinnamon stick (1)
- ❖ Lemon (1, sliced thinly)
- ❖ Boiling water (6 cups)

Directions:
1. In a large teapot, place the tea leaves, lemon slices and cinnamon stick.
2. Pour hot water over the ingredients and immediately cover the teapot.
3. Set aside for about 5 minutes to steep.
4. Strain the tea in mugs and serve immediately.

Lemony Black Coffee

Serving|1 Time|9 minutes
Nutritional Content (per serving):
| 24 Fat| 0g Protein| 0.6g Carbs| 6.1g Fiber| 0g

Ingredients:
- ❖ Coffee powder (¼ teaspoon)
- ❖ Fresh lemon juice (1 teaspoon)
- ❖ Filtered water (1¼ cups)
- ❖ Honey (1 teaspoon)

Directions:
1. In a small pan, add the water and coffee powder and bring to boil.
2. Cook for about 1 minute.
3. Remove the coffee from heat and pour into a serving mug.
4. Add the honey and lemon juice and stir until dissolved
5. Serve hot.

Chicken Bones Broth

Servings|10   Time|6 hours
Nutritional Content (per serving):
Cal| 141   Fat| 2.6g   Protein| 25.8g   Carbs| 0.6g   Fiber| 0.1g

Ingredients:

- ❖ Chicken bones (4 pounds)
- ❖ Filtered water (10 cups)
- ❖ Lemon, quartered (1)
- ❖ Ground turmeric (3 teaspoons)
- ❖ Sea salt, as required
- ❖ Apple cider vinegar (2 tablespoons)
- ❖ Bay leaves (3)
- ❖ Black peppercorns (2 tablespoons)

Directions:

1. Preheat your oven to 400 degrees F.
2. Arrange the bones onto a large baking sheet and sprinkle with salt.
3. Roast for approximately 45 minutes.
4. Remove from the oven and transfer the bones into a large pan.
5. Add in the remaining ingredients and stir to combine.
6. Place the pan over medium-high heat and bring to a boil.
7. Now adjust the heat to low and simmer, covered for about 4-5 hours, skimming the foam from the surface occasionally.
8. Through a fine-mesh sieve, strain the broth into a large bowl.
9. Serve hot.

Chicken Bones & Veggie Broth

Servings|12   Time|12 hours 40 minutes
Nutritional Content (per serving):
Cal| 67   Fat| 4.1g   Protein| 5.7g   Carbs| 2g   Fiber| 0.5g

Ingredients:
- Extra-virgin olive oil (3 tablespoons)
- Large carrots (2, peeled and chopped roughly)
- Whole cloves (2)
- Warm water, as required
- Chicken bones (2½ pounds)
- Celery stalks (4, chopped roughly)
- Bay leaf (1)
- Black peppercorns (1 tablespoon)
- Apple cider vinegar (1 tablespoon)

Directions:
1. In a Dutch oven, heat the oil over medium-high heat and sear the bones or about 3-5 minutes or until browned.
2. With a slotted spoon, transfer the bones into a bowl.
3. In the same pan, add the celery stalks and carrots and cook for about 15 minutes, stirring occasionally.
4. Add browned bones, bay leaf, black peppercorns, cloves and vinegar and stir to combine.
5. Add the enough warm water to cover the bones mixture completely and bring to a gentle boil.
6. Now adjust the heat to low and simmer, covered for about 8-10 hours, skimming the foam from the surface occasionally.
7. Through a fine-mesh sieve, strain the broth into a large bowl.
8. Serve hot.

Chicken & Veggie Broth

Servings|8   Time|2 hours 20 minutes
Nutritional Content (per serving):
Cal| 275   Fat| 5.2g   Protein| 49.7g   Carbs| 4.3g   Fiber| 1.2g

Ingredients:
- ❖ Whole chicken (3-pound, cut into pieces)
- ❖ Celery stalks with leaves (4, cut into 2-inch pieces)
- ❖ Sea salt, as required
- ❖ Medium carrots (5, peeled and cut into 2-inch pieces)
- ❖ Fresh thyme sprigs (6)
- ❖ Fresh parsley sprigs (6)
- ❖ Filtered water (9 cups)

Directions:
1. In a large Dutch oven, add all the ingredients over medium-high heat and bring to a boil.
2. Now adjust the heat to medium-low and simmer, covered for about 2 hours, skimming the foam from the surface occasionally.
3. Through a fine-mesh sieve, strain the broth into a large bowl.
4. Serve hot.

Fish Broth

Servings|6   Time|12¼ hours
Nutritional Content (per serving):
Cal| 75   Fat| 1.7g   Protein| 13.4g   Carbs| 0.1g   Fiber| 0g

Ingredients:
- ❖ Filtered water (12 cups)
- ❖ Apple cider vinegar (¼ cup)
- ❖ Sea salt, as required
- ❖ Non-oily fish carcasses and heads (2 pounds)

Directions:
1. In a large heavy-bottomed saucepan, add all the ingredients over medium-high heat.
2. Add enough water to cover the veggie mixture and bring to a boil.
3. Now adjust the heat to low and simmer, covered for about 10-12 hours, skimming the foam from the surface occasionally.
4. Through a fine-mesh sieve, strain the broth into a large bowl.
5. Serve hot.

Fish & Veggie Broth

Servings|8   Time|2 hours 40 minutes
Nutritional Content (per serving):
Cal| 113   Fat| 5.2g   Protein| 13.7g   Carbs| 2.5g   Fiber| 0.7g

Ingredients:

- Non-oily fish carcasses and heads 5-7 pounds)
- Carrots (3, scrubbed and chopped roughly)
- Black peppercorns (1½ tablespoons)
- Fresh thyme stems (4)
- Olive oil (2 tablespoons)
- Celery stalks (2, chopped roughly)
- Bay leaf (1)
- Whole cloves (2)
- Bunch fresh parsley (1)

Directions:

1. In a large pan, heat the oil over medium-low heat and cook the carrots and celery for about 20 minutes, stirring occasionally.
2. Add the fish bones and enough water to cover and stir to combine.
3. Now adjust the heat to medium-high and bring to a boil.
4. Now adjust the heat to low and simmer, covered for about 1-2 hours, skimming the foam from the surface occasionally.
5. Through a fine-mesh sieve, strain the broth into a large bowl.
6. Serve hot.

Veggie Broth

Servings|10   Time|2 hours 20 minutes
Nutritional Content (per serving):
Cal| 82   Fat| 0.2g   Protein| 1.9g   Carbs| 19g   Fiber| 3.7g

Ingredients:

- Carrots (4, peeled and chopped roughly)
- Large potatoes (2, peeled and chopped roughly)
- Large bunch fresh parsley (1)
- Fresh ginger (1-inch piece)
- Parsnips (3, peeled and chopped roughly)
- Celery stalks (4, chopped roughly)
- Medium beet (1, trimmed and chopped roughly0
- Water, as required

Directions:

1. In a large saucepan, add all the ingredients over medium-high heat.
2. Add enough water to cover the veggie mixture and bring to a boil.
3. Now adjust the heat to low and simmer, covered for about 2-3 hours.
4. Through a fine-mesh sieve, strain the broth into a large bowl.
5. Serve hot.

Mushroom, Cauliflower & Cabbage Broth

Servings|3   Time|1 hour
Nutritional Content (per serving):
Cal| 141   Fat| 5g   Protein| 5g   Carbs| 22g   Fiber| 7g

Ingredients:

- Large yellow onion (1)
- celery stalks (1 cup, chopped)
- carrots (2, diced or cubed)
- French beans (10)
- cabbage (½, diced)
- celery leaves (1 to 2 stalks)
- mushrooms (1½ cup, sliced)
- cauliflower (8 florets)
- garlic (1 teaspoon, chopped)
- ginger (1 teaspoon, chopped)
- oil (1 tablespoon)
- Scallions (1 stalk)
- pepper (½ teaspoon crushed)

Directions:

1. Transfer all your ingredients to your stockpot. Top with enough water to cover then allow to slowly come to a boil on high heat.
2. Switch to low heat and simmer for 50 minutes.
3. Carefully pour the mixture through a fine mesh strainer into a large bowl. Mash the veggies well to extract all their juices.
4. Taste and season with salt. Enjoy.

Indian Inspired Vegetable stock

Servings|3   Time|1 hour
Nutritional Content (per serving):
Cal| 103   Fat| 0.2g   Protein| 2.2g   Carbs| 23.3g   Fiber| 3.1g

Ingredients:

- Onions (3/4 cup, roughly chopped)
- Carrot (3/4 cup, roughly chopped)
- Tomatoes (3/4 cup, roughly chopped)
- Potatoes (¾ cup, roughly chopped)
- Turmeric (1 teaspoon)
- salt to taste

Directions:

1. Transfer your ingredients to your stockpot. Top with enough water to cover then allow to slowly come to a boil on high heat.
2. Switch to low heat and simmer for 11 minutes.
3. Carefully pour the mixture through a fine mesh strainer into a large bowl. Taste and season with salt.
4. Serve hot. Enjoy!

Beef Bone Broth

Servings|8   Time|12¼ hours
Nutritional Content (per serving):
Cal| 69   Fat| 4g   Protein| 6g   Carbs| 1g   Fiber| 0.1g

Ingredients:

- beef bones (2 pounds)
- onion (1, chopped in quarters)
- celery stalks (2, chopped in half)
- carrots (2, chopped in half)
- garlic cloves (3, whole)
- bay leaves (2)
- apple cider vinegar (2 Tablespoons)
- salt (1 Tablespoon)
- peppercorns (½ tablespoon)
- Filtered water (enough to cover bones)

Directions:

1. Transfer the bones and vegetables to your stockpot. Top with enough water to cover then allow to slowly come to a boil on high heat.
2. Switch to low heat and simmer for at least 2 hours and up to 12 hours. (The longer it cooks, the more flavor you will get.)
3. Carefully pour the mixture through a fine mesh strainer into a large bowl. Taste and season with salt.

Ginger, Mushroom & Cauliflower Broth

Servings|3   Time|1 hour
Nutritional Content (per serving):
Cal| 141   Fat| 5g   Protein| 5g   Carbs| 22g   Fiber| 7g

Ingredients:

- ❖ Large yellow onion (1)
- ❖ celery stalks (1 cup, chopped)
- ❖ carrots (2, diced or cubed)
- ❖ 10 French beans
- ❖ 1 ginger root, peeled and diced or grated
- ❖ 1 to 2 stalks celery leaves or cilantro leaves
- ❖ Mushrooms (1½ cups, sliced)
- ❖ 8 florets cauliflower
- ❖ 1 teaspoon garlic chopped
- ❖ Oil (1 tablespoon)
- ❖ 1 stalk spring onion greens or Scallions
- ❖ ½ teaspoon crushed pepper or Ground pepper

Directions:

1. Transfer your ingredients to your stockpot. Top with enough water to cover then allow to slowly come to a boil on high heat.
2. Switch to low heat and simmer for at least 50 minutes on low hat.
3. Carefully pour the mixture through a fine mesh strainer into a large bowl. Taste and season with salt.
4. Serve hot. Enjoy!

Fish & Mushroom Broth

Servings|32   Time|1 hour
Nutritional Content (per serving):
Cal| 29   Fat| 1g   Protein| 1g   Carbs| 2g   Fiber| 1g

Ingredients:

- olive oil (3 tablespoons)
- onion (1 Large, chopped)
- carrot (1 Large, chopped)
- fennel bulb (1, chopped, optional)
- celery stalks (3, chopped)
- Salt
- white wine (2 cups)
- fish bones and heads (2 to 5 pounds)
- mushrooms (A handful of dried, optional)
- bay leaves (2 to 4)
- 1-star anise pod (optional)
- Thyme (1 to 2 teaspoons dried or Fresh)
- kombu kelp (3 or 4 pieces of dried, optional)
- Chopped fronds from the fennel bulb

Directions:

1. Transfer the bones and vegetables to your stockpot. Top with enough water to cover then allow to slowly come to a boil on high heat.
2. Switch to low heat and simmer for 45 mins.
3. Carefully pour the mixture through a fine mesh strainer into a large bowl. Taste and season with salt.
4. Serve hot. Enjoy!

Clear Pumpkin Broth

Servings|6   Time|45 minutes
Nutritional Content (per serving):
Cal| 216   Fat| 1g   Protein| 8g   Carbs| 37g   Fiber| 4g

Ingredients:
- instant dashi powder (3 teaspoons)
- sake or dry sherry (1 cup)
- mirin (2 tablespoons)
- soy sauce (1 cup)
- sugar (2 tablespoons)
- water (6 cups)
- ginger (2 tablespoons, minced)
- potatoes (2 cups, peeled and diced)
- kabocha (3 cups, peeled and diced)
- carrot (1, peeled and diced)
- onion (1, diced)
- Scallions (½ cup, chopped)

Directions:
1. Transfer the bones and vegetables to your stockpot. Top with enough water to cover then allow to slowly come to a boil on high heat.
2. Switch to low heat and simmer for at least 30 minutes
3. Carefully pour the mixture through a fine mesh strainer into a large bowl. Taste and season with salt.

Pork Stock

Servings|8   Time|12¼ hours
Nutritional Content (per serving):
Cal| 69   Fat| 4g   Protein| 6g   Carbs| 1g   Fiber| 0.1g

Ingredients:
- pork bones (2 Pounds, roasted)
- onion (1, chopped in quarters)
- celery stalks (2, chopped in half)
- carrots (2, chopped in half)
- garlic cloves (3, whole)
- bay leaves (2)
- apple cider vinegar (2 Tablespoons)
- salt (1 Tablespoon)
- peppercorns (1/2 Tablespoon)
- Filtered water (enough to cover bones)

Directions:
1. Transfer the bones and vegetables to your stockpot. Top with enough water to cover then allow to slowly come to a boil on high heat.
2. Switch to low heat and simmer for 12 hours on low. (The longer it cooks, the more flavor you will get.)
3. Carefully pour the mixture through a fine mesh strainer into a large bowl. Taste and season with salt.
4. Serve hot. Enjoy!

Slow Cooker Pork Bone Broth

Servings|12   Time|24¼ hours + roasting time
Nutritional Content (per serving):
Cal| 65   Fat| 2g   Protein| 6g   Carbs| 7g   Fiber| 4g

Ingredients:

- ❖ pork bones (2 pounds – roasted)
- ❖ onion (½ chopped)
- ❖ carrots (2 Medium chopped)
- ❖ celery (1 stalk chopped)
- ❖ garlic whole (2 cloves)
- ❖ bay leaf (1)
- ❖ sea salt (1 tablespoon)
- ❖ peppercorns (1 teaspoon)
- ❖ Apple Cider Vinegar (¼ cup)
- ❖ Filtered water

Directions:

1. Transfer your ingredients to your slow cooker. Top with enough water to cover then allow to slowly come to a boil on high heat.
2. Switch to low heat and simmer for at least 24 hours on low. (The longer it cooks, the more flavor you will get.)
3. Carefully pour the mixture through a fine mesh strainer into a large bowl. Taste and season with salt.
4. Serve hot. Enjoy!

Lemon Gelatin

Servings|8   Time|10 minutes
Nutritional Content (per serving)
Cal| 18   Fat| 0.3g   Protein| 2.5g   Carbs| 0.7g   Fiber| 0.1g

Ingredients:

- Grass-fed gelatin powder (3 tablespoons)
- Boiling water (1½ cups)
- Stevia extract (2 teaspoons)
- Cold water (3 cups, divided)
- Fresh lemon juice (1 cup plus 2 tablespoons)

Directions:

1. In a bowl, soak the gelatin in (1½ cups) of cold water. Set aside for about 5 minutes.
2. Add boiling water and stir until gelatin is dissolved.
3. Add the remaining cold water, lemon juice and stevia extract and stir until dissolved completely.
4. Divide the mixture into 2 baking dishes and refrigerate until set before serving.

Tangerine Gelatin

Servings|4   Time|10 minutes
Nutritional Content (per serving):
Cal| 13   Fat| 0g   Protein| 2.8g   Carbs| 0.4g   Fiber| 0g

Ingredients:

- Grass-fed tangerine gelatin powder (1 tablespoon)
- Boiling water (2¼ cups)

Directions:

1. In a large bowl, add the gelatin and boiling water and stir until dissolved completely.
2. Divide in serving bowls and refrigerate until set completely before serving.

Grapefruit Gelatin

Servings|4 Time|15 minutes
Nutritional Content (per serving):
Cal| 94   Fat| 0.1g   Protein| 2g   Carbs| 23.3   Fiber| 0.8g

Ingredients:
- Grass-fed gelatin powder (1 tablespoon)
- Fresh grapefruit juice (1¼ cups)
- Cold water (¾ cup, divided)
- Honey (¼ cup)
- Pinch of sea salt

Directions:
1. In a bowl, soak the gelatin in ¼ cup of cold water. Set aside.
2. In a Small saucepan, add the remaining water and honey over medium heat and bring to a boil.
3. Simmer for about 3 minutes or until honey is dissolved completely.
4. Remove from the heat and stir in the soaked gelatin until dissolved completely.
5. Set aside at room temperature to cool completely.
6. After cooling, stir in the grapefruit juice and salt.
7. Transfer the mixture into serving bowls and refrigerate for about 4 hours or until set.

Grape Gelatin

Servings|8 Time|10 minutes
Nutritional Content (per serving):
Cal| 15   Fat| 0g   Protein| 0.9g   Carbs| 2.8g   Fiber| 0g

Ingredients:
- Grass-fed gelatin powder (1 tablespoon)
- Hot water (¼ cup)
- Cold water (¼ cup)
- Fresh grape juice (1 cup)

Directions:
1. In a bowl, soak the gelatin in cold water. Set aside for about 5 minutes.
2. Add the hot water and mix well. Set aside for about 1-2 minutes.
3. Add the grape juice and mix well.
4. Divide in serving bowls and refrigerate until set completely before serving.

Apple Gelatin

Servings|6   Time|10 minutes
Nutritional Content (per serving)
Cal| 37   Fat| 0.1g   Protein| 1.1g   Carbs| 8.2g   Fiber| 0.2g

Ingredients:
- Grass-fed gelatin powder (1 tablespoon)
- Boiling water (¼ cup)
- Warm fresh apple juice (1¾ cups)
- Fresh lemon juice (1-2 drops)

Directions:
1. In a medium bowl, add in the gelatin powder.
2. Add just enough warm apple juice to cover the gelatin and stir well.
3. Set aside for about 2-3 minutes or until it forms a thick syrup.
4. Add the boiling water and stir until gelatin is dissolved completely.
5. Add the remaining apple juice and lemon juice and stir well.
6. Transfer the mixture into a parchment paper-lined baking dish and refrigerate for 2 hours or until the top is firm before serving.

Peach Gelatin

Servings|10   Time|15 minutes
Nutritional Content (per serving):
Cal| 66   Fat| 0g   Protein| 1.2g   Carbs| 15.5g   Fiber| 0g

Ingredients:
- Grass-fed gelatin powder (2 tablespoons)
- Honey (2 tablespoons)
- Fresh peach juice (4½ cups, divided)

Directions:
1. In a bowl, soak the gelatin in ½ cup of juice. Set aside for about 5 minutes.
2. In a medium pan, add the remaining juice over medium heat and bring to a gentle boil.
3. Remove from the heat and stir in honey.
4. Add the gelatin mixture and stir until dissolved.
5. Transfer the mixture into a large baking dish and refrigerate until set completely before serving.

Cinnamon Gelatin

Servings|2 Time|15 minutes
Nutritional Content (per serving):
Cal| 76   Fat| 0g   Protein| 3.7g   Carbs| 17.3g   Fiber| 0g

Ingredients:
- ❖ Filtered water (1 cup)
- ❖ Cinnamon stick (1)
- ❖ Grass-fed gelatin powder (2 teaspoons)
- ❖ Honey (2 tablespoons)

Directions:
1. In a small pan, add the water over medium heat and bring to a boil.
2. Add in the cinnamon stick and turn off the heat.
3. Immediately, cover the pan and steep for 3 minutes.
4. Add the gelatin and beat until well combined.
5. Transfer the mixture into a baking dish and set aside to cool for about 2 hours.
6. Refrigerate to set before serving.

Homemade Banana Apple Juice

Servings|2   Time|10 minutes
Nutritional Content (per serving):
Cal| 132   Fat| 2g   Protein| 4g   Carbs| 27g   Fiber| 3g

Ingredients:
- ❖ Bananas (2, peeled, sliced)
- ❖ Apple (1/2, peeled, cored and chopped)
- ❖ Honey (1 tablespoon)
- ❖ Water (1½ cups)

Directions:
1. Add all your ingredients into your blender, and blend.
2. Set a fine mesh strainer a bowl. Before transferring your juice into the strainer.
3. Gently press the pulp to extract all possible liquid then discard pulp.
4. Serve over ice. Enjoy!

Sweet Detox Juice

Servings|2   Time|10 minutes
Nutritional Content (per serving):
Cal| 209   Fat| 2g   Protein| 12g   Carbs| 17.3g   Fiber| 17g

Ingredients:
- ❖ baby spinach (2 cups, chopped)
- ❖ parsley (1 handful, chopped)
- ❖ apple (1, green, peeled, cored, seeded, sliced0
- ❖ cucumber (1 Large English, seeded, chopped)
- ❖ ginger (1-inch, peeled)
- ❖ lemon (1, juiced)

Directions:
1. Add all your ingredients into your blender, and blend.
2. Set a fine mesh strainer a bowl. Before transferring your juice into the strainer.
3. Gently press the pulp to extract all possible liquid then discard pulp.
4. Serve over ice. Enjoy!

Pineapple Ginger Juice

Servings|7   Time|10 minutes
Nutritional Content (per serving):
Cal| 71   Fat| 1g   Protein| 1g   Carbs| 20g   Fiber| 3g

Ingredients:
- pineapple (10 cups, chopped)
- water (6 cups)
- Apples (3, Fuji, chopped)
- ginger (4-inch root, peeled, chopped)
- lemon juice (1/4 cup)
- sugar (1/4 cup)

Directions:
1. Add all your ingredients into your blender, and blend.
2. Set a fine mesh strainer a bowl. Before transferring your juice into the strainer.
3. Gently press the pulp to extract all possible liquid then discard pulp.
4. Serve over ice. Enjoy!

Tropical Fruit Punch

Servings|4   Time|10 minutes
Nutritional Content (per serving):
Cal| 247   Fat| 1g   Protein| 3g   Carbs| 65g   Fiber| 10g

Ingredients:
- Pineapple (1, peeled, cored, sliced)
- Apples (2, peeled, cored, quartered)
- Oranges (2, juiced)
- Pears (2, peeled, seeded, quartered)
- Lime (1, juiced)
- Water (2 cups)

Directions:
   Add all your ingredients into your blender, and blend.
1. Set a fine mesh strainer a bowl. Before transferring your juice into the strainer.
2. Gently press the pulp to extract all possible liquid then discard pulp.
3. Serve over ice. Enjoy!

Carrot Orange Juice

Servings|2   Time|10 minutes
Nutritional Content (per serving):
Cal| 111   Fat| 1g   Protein| 2g   Carbs| 24g   Fiber| 1g

Ingredients:
- Tomato (1, yellow, medium), cut into wedges
- Orange (1, peeled, quartered)
- Apple (1, peeled, cored, chopped)
- Carrots (4, jumbo, peeled, chopped)
- Water (2 cups)

Directions:
1. Add all your ingredients into your blender, and blend.
2. Set a fine mesh strainer a bowl. Before transferring your juice into the strainer.
3. Gently press the pulp to extract all possible liquid then discard pulp.
4. Serve over ice. Enjoy!

Strawberry Apple Juice

Servings|1   Time|5 minutes
Nutritional Content (per serving):
Cal| 245   Fat| 5g   Protein| 4g   Carbs| 52g   Fiber| 7g

Ingredients:
- Strawberries (2 cups, tops removed)
- Apple (1, red, peeled, seeded, cored, chopped)
- Chia seeds (1 tablespoon)
- Water (1 cup)

Directions:
1. Add all your ingredients into your blender, and blend.
2. Set a fine mesh strainer a bowl. Before transferring your juice into the strainer.
3. Gently press the pulp to extract all possible liquid then discard pulp.
4. Add in your chia seeds then leave to sit for at least 5 minutes.
5. Serve over ice. Enjoy!

Autumn Energizer Juice

Servings|2   Time|10 minutes
Nutritional Content (per serving):
Cal| 170   Fat| 3g   Protein| 4g   Carbs| 33g   Fiber| 9g

Ingredients:

- Pears (2, peeled, seeded, chopped)
- Apples (2, Ambrosia, peeled, cored, chopped)
- Apples (2, Granny Smith, peeled, cored, chopped)
- Mandarins (2, juiced)
- sweet potato (2 cups, peeled, chopped)
- cape gooseberries (1 pint)
- Ginger (2-inch root, peeled)

Directions:

1. Add all your ingredients into your blender, and blend.
2. Set a fine mesh strainer a bowl. Before transferring your juice into the strainer.
3. Gently press the pulp to extract all possible liquid then discard pulp.
4. Serve over ice. Enjoy!

Phase: 2- Low-Residue Recipes

Breakfast Recipes

Carrot, Greens & Celery Juice

Servings|2   Time|10 minutes
Nutritional Content (per serving):
Cal| 36   Fat| 0.4g   Protein| 2.5g   Carbs| 7.1g   Fiber| 2.7g

Ingredients:

- Fresh spinach (3 cups)
- Large carrot (1, peeled and chopped roughly)
- lemon (1)
- Fresh arugula (3 cups)
- celery stalks (2)
- Fresh ginger (1-inch piece, peeled)

Directions:

1. Add all ingredients into a juicer and extract the juice according to the manufacturer's method.
2. Through a cheesecloth-lined strainer, strain the juice and transfer into 2 glasses.
3. Serve immediately.

Ripe Plantain Bran Muffins

Servings|12 Time|30 minutes
Nutritional Content (per serving):
Cal| 325   Fat| 19g   Protein| 3g   Carbs| 37g   Fiber| 2g

Ingredients:

- Refined Cereal (1 1/2 cups)
- Milk (2/3 cup, low fat)
- Eggs (4, Large, lightly beaten)
- Canola oil (1/4 cup)
- Ripe plantain (2, Medium, mashed, 1 cup)
- Brown sugar (1/2 cup)
- Refined flour (1 cup, white)
- Baking powder (2 teaspoons)
- Salt (1/2 teaspoon)

Directions:

1. Preheat oven to 400 degrees F. In a large bowl, combine bran cereal and milk and set aside.
2. Add eggs and oil; stir in brown sugar and mashed ripe plantain. In another bowl, combine salt, flour, and baking powder.
3. Add the dry ingredients into the ripe plantain mixture, stir until combined.
4. Pour batter evenly into a paper-lined muffin tins; Bake 18 minutes or until golden-brown and firm. Allow to cool prior to serving.

Easy Breakfast Bran Muffins

Servings|10 Time|30 minutes
Nutritional Content (per serving):
Cal| 440   Fat| 20g   Protein| 9g   Carbs| 57g   Fiber| 3g

Ingredients:

- Refined cereal (2 cups)
- Brown sugar (1/2 cup)
- Butter (1/2 cup)
- Eggs (2)
- Buttermilk (1/2 quart)

- White flour (2 1/2 cups, refined)
- Baking soda (2 1/2 teaspoon)
- Salt (1/2 teaspoon)

Directions:

1. Preheat oven to 400 degrees F. Soak 1 cup cereal in 1 cup boiling water and set aside.
2. In a mixer, cream sugar and butter together until it is fully mixed. Add each egg separate and beat until fluffy. Add buttermilk and soaked cereal mixture.
3. In another bowl, combine salt, flour and baking soda. Add the flour mixture into the batter and ensure not to over mix.
4. Add in remaining 1 cup of cereal. Pour batter evenly into 10 greased or paper-lined muffin tins. Bake 15-20 minutes. Allow to cool prior to serving.

Apple Oatmeal

Servings|1 Time|9 minutes
Nutritional Content (per serving):
Cal| 295   Fat| 7g   Protein| 13g   Carbs| 47g   Fiber| 5g

Ingredients:
- ❖ Instant oatmeal (1/2 cup)
- ❖ milk or water (3/4 cup)
- ❖ apples (1/2 cup, peeled, cooked pureed)
- ❖ brown sugar (1 teaspoon)

Directions:
1. In a microwave-safe bowl, mix oats, milk or water and apples. Cook in microwave on high for 45 seconds.
2. Stir and microwave for another 30 seconds. Sprinkle with brown sugar and add a splash of milk.

Breakfast Burrito Wraps

Servings|1 Time|30 minutes
Nutritional Content (per serving):
Cal| 355   Fat| 2g   Protein| 23g   Carbs| 14g   Fiber| 4g

Ingredients:
- ❖ Olive oil (1 tablespoon, extra virgin)
- ❖ Turkey bacon (2 slices)
- ❖ Green bell peppers (1/4 cup, seeded and chopped)
- ❖ Eggs (2, beaten)
- ❖ Milk (2 tablespoons)
- ❖ Salt (1/4 teaspoon)
- ❖ Monterrey Jack cheese (2 tablespoons, low- fat, grated)
- ❖ Tortilla (1, white)

Directions:
1. In a small non-stick pan, heat olive oil on Medium heat and cook turkey about 2 minutes until slightly crispy.
2. Add bell peppers and continue to cook until warmed through. In a Small bowl beat together egg with milk and salt.
3. Gently stir in your eggs until almost cooked through. Turn the heat down then add the cheese.
4. Cover and continue to cook until cheese have completely melted. Place the mixture on the tortilla and roll it into a burrito.

Zucchini Omelet

Servings|4   Time|30 minutes
Nutritional Content (per serving):
Cal| 295   Fat| 10g   Protein| 6g   Carbs| 14g   Fiber| 2g

Ingredients:

- Olive oil (2 tablespoons, extra virgin)
- Zucchini (1, medium, seeded, cubed)
- Tomato (1/2 medium, seeded, chopped)
- Eggs (4, large)
- Milk (1/4 cup)
- Salt (1 teaspoon)
- English muffins (4, whole wheat)

Directions:
1. In a large non-stick pan, heat olive oil over moderate heat. Add Zucchini and tomato.
2. Cook vegetables for 5-10 minutes or until they are soft. In a separate bowl, mix eggs and milk and salt.
3. Add egg mixture to pan and stir to cook through, about 5 minutes. Serve with white English muffins.

Coconut Chia Seed Pudding

Servings|2   Time|10 minutes
Nutritional Content (per serving):
Cal| 223   Fat| 12g   Protein| 10g   Carbs| 18g   Fiber| 2g

Ingredients:

- Chia seeds (6 tablespoons)
- Coconut milk (2 cups, unsweetened)
- Blueberries for topping

Directions:
1. Combine the chia seeds and milk and mix well. Refrigerate overnight. Stir in the berries and serve.

Spiced Oatmeal

Servings|1   Time|7 minutes
Nutritional Content (per serving):
Cal| 467   Fat| 11g   Protein| 6g   Carbs| 33g   Fiber| 4g

Ingredients:
- Quick oats (1/3 cup)
- Banana (1/2)
- Ginger (1/4 teaspoon, ground)
- Cinnamon (1/8 teaspoon, ground)
- Small sprinkle nutmeg ground
- Small sprinkle cloves ground
- almond butte (1 tablespoon)

Directions:
1. Combine the oats and water. Microwave for 45 seconds, then stir and cook for another 30-45 seconds.
2. Stir in the spices and drizzle on the almond butter before serving.

Breakfast Cereal

Servings|4   Time|10 minutes
Nutritional Content (per serving):
Cal| 228   Fat| 3.8g   Protein| 12g   Carbs| 43g   Fiber| 6g

Ingredients:
- old fashioned oatmeal (3 cups, cooked)
- quinoa (3 cups, cooked)
- 4 cups banana, peeled, chopped

Directions:
1. Combine the oatmeal and quinoa and mix well. Evenly divide into four bowls and top with the bananas before serving.

Sweet Potato with Sausage & Spinach

Servings|4   Time|20 minutes
Nutritional Content (per serving):
Cal| 544   Fat| 2g   Protein| 11g   Carbs| 65g   Fiber| 2g

Ingredients:
- sweet potatoes (4 small, chopped)
- apples (2, cored and chopped)
- 1 clove garlic (minced)
- sausage (1 pound, ground)
- spinach (10 ounces chopped)
- Salt & pepper

Directions:
1. Brown the sausage until no pink remains. Add the remaining ingredients.
2. Cook for an additional 5-6 minutes, or until the spinach and apples are tender. Season to taste and serve hot.

Cajun Omelet

Servings|2   Time|13 minutes
Nutritional Content (per serving):
Cal| 467   Fat| 14g   Protein| 3g   Carbs| 11g   Fiber| 2g

Ingredients:
- sausage (1/4 pound, spicy)
- mushrooms (1/3 cup, sliced)
- onion (1/2, diced eggs (4 Large)
- ½ Medium bell pepper, chopped
- water (2 tablespoons)
- cooking Fat
- 1 pinch cayenne pepper (optional)
- Sea salt & Fresh pepper to taste

Directions:
1. Brown the sausage in a medium saucepan until cooked through. Add the mushrooms, onion and bell pepper and cook for another 3-5 minutes, or until tender.
2. Meanwhile, whisk together the eggs, water, mustard and spices. Season with the salt and pepper.
3. Top with your eggs over then reduce to a low heat. Cook until the top is nearly set and then fold the omelet in half and cover. Cook for another minute before serving hot.

Strawberry Cashew Chia Pudding

Servings|2   Time|10 minutes
Nutritional Content (per serving):
Cal| 223   Fat| 12g   Protein| 10g   Carbs| 18g   Fiber| 2g

Ingredients:
- ❖ chia seeds (6 tablespoons)
- ❖ cashew milk (2 cups, unsweetened)
- ❖ Strawberries, for topping

Directions:
1. Combine the chia seeds and milk and mix well. Refrigerate overnight. Stir in the berries and serve.

Peanut Butter Banana Oatmeal

Servings|1   Time|10 minutes
Nutritional Content (per serving):
Cal| 645   Fat| 32g   Protein| 26g   Carbs| 65g   Fiber| 5g

Ingredients:
- ❖ quick oats (1/3 cup)
- ❖ cinnamon (1/4 teaspoon (optional)
- ❖ banana (1/2, sliced)
- ❖ peanut butter (1 tablespoon, unsweetened)

Directions:
1. Combine all ingredients in a bowl with a lid. Refrigerate.

Overnight Peach Oatmeal

Servings|2 Time|10 minutes
Nutritional Content (per serving):
Cal| 282   Fat| 32g   Protein| 26g   Carbs| 65g   Fiber| 5g

Ingredients:
- oats (½ cup, old fashioned)
- Greek yogurt (½ cup, plain)
- Vanilla (½ teaspoon)
- banana (1 medium, peeled, chopped)
- skim milk (2/3 cup)
- chia seeds (1 tablespoon)
- peach (½ cup, peeled, diced)

Directions:
1. Combine the oats, milk, yogurt, chia seeds and vanilla in a bowl with a lid.
2. Refrigerate for 12 hours.
3. Top with fruit before serving.

Carrot, Tomato & Celery Juice

Servings|3   Time|10 minutes
Nutritional Content (per serving):
Cal| 62   Fat| 0.5g   Protein| 2.5g   Carbs| 13.7g   Fiber| 4g

Ingredients:
- Tomatoes (6)
- Large celery stalk (1)
- Pinch of sea salt and ground black pepper
- Carrots (2, peeled)
- Filtered water (¼ cup)
- 3-4 ice cubes

Directions:
1. Place all the ingredients in a blender and pulse until well combined.
2. Through a cheesecloth-lined strainer, strain the juice and transfer into 3 glasses.
3. Serve immediately.

Tomato & Basil Scramble

Servings|2   Time|15 minutes
Nutritional Content (per serving):
Cal| 195   Fat| 15.9g   Protein| 11.6g   Carbs| 2.6g   Fiber| 0.7g

Ingredients:
- Eggs (4)
- Sea salt and ground black pepper, as required
- Tomatoes (½ cup, peeled, seeded and chopped)
- Red pepper flakes (¼ teaspoon, crushed)
- Fresh basil (¼ cup, chopped)
- Olive oil (1 tablespoon)

Directions:
1. In a bowl, add eggs, red pepper flakes, salt and black pepper and beat well.
2. Add the basil and tomatoes and stir to combine.
3. In a large non-stick skillet, heat the oil over medium-high heat.
4. Add the egg mixture and cook for about 3-5 minutes, stirring continuously.
5. Serve immediately.

Salmon & Spinach Scramble

Servings|3   Time|17 minutes
Nutritional Content (per serving):
Cal| 179   Fat| 12.9g   Protein| 15.3g   Carbs| 1.2g   Fiber| 0.4g

Ingredients:
- Fresh spinach (2 cups, chopped finely)
- Sea salt and ground black pepper, as required
- Olive oil (1 tablespoon)
- Cooked salmon (½ cup, chopped finely)
- Eggs (4, beaten)

Directions:
1. In a skillet, heat the oil over high heat and cook the spinach with black pepper for about 2 minutes.
2. Stir in the salmon and immediately adjust the heat to medium.
3. Add the eggs and cook for about 3-4 minutes, stirring frequently.
4. Serve immediately.

Mushroom & Bell Pepper Omelet

Servings|4   Time|35 minutes
Nutritional Content (per serving):
Cal| 125   Fat| 7.8g   Protein| 10.8g   Carbs| 3.1g   Fiber| 0.2g

Ingredients:
- Large eggs (6)
- Low-fat milk (½ cup)
- Fresh mushrooms (1/3 cup, sliced)
- Fresh chives (1 teaspoon, minced)
- Sea salt and ground black pepper, as required
- Red bell pepper (1/3 cup, seeded and chopped)

Directions:
1. Preheat your oven to 350 degrees F. Lightly grease a pie dish.
2. In a bowl, add the eggs, salt, black pepper and milk and beat until well combined.
3. In another bowl, mix together the bell pepper and mushrooms.
4. Transfer the egg mixture into the prepared pie dish evenly.
5. Top with vegetable mixture evenly and sprinkle with chives evenly.
6. Bake for approximately 20-25 minutes.
7. Remove from the oven and set aside for about 5 minutes.
8. With a knife, cut into equal-sized wedges and serve.

Avocado & Scallion Frittata

Servings|6   Time|27 minutes
Nutritional Content (per serving):
Cal| 207   Fat| 16.6g   Protein| 10.8g   Carbs| 5.1g   Fiber| 2.4g

Ingredients:

- ❖ Eggs (8, beaten well)
- ❖ Sea salt and ground black pepper, as required
- ❖ Part-skim mozzarella cheese (½ cup, grated)
- ❖ Olive oil (2 teaspoons)
- ❖ Low-fat milk (½ cup)
- ❖ Feta cheese (2 ounces, crumbled)
- ❖ Scallion (¼ cup, sliced)
- ❖ Large avocado (1, peeled, pitted and sliced lengthwise)

Directions:

1. Preheat the broiler of oven. Arrange the oven rack about 4-5-inch from the heating element.
2. In a bowl, add the eggs, milk, salt and black pepper and beat until well combined.
3. In a heavy oven-proof frying skillet, heat the oil over medium-low heat.
4. Add the eggs and cook for about 2 minutes.
5. Add the mozzarella and scallion and cook for about 5 minutes.
6. Arrange the avocado slices over egg mixture and sprinkle with the feta cheese.
7. With ae lid, cover the skillet and cook about 3 minutes.
8. Remove lid and transfer the skillet into the oven.
9. Broil for about 2 minutes.
10. Remove from the oven and set aside for about 5 minutes.
11. With a knife, cut into equal-sized wedges and serve.

Green Veggies Quiche

Servings|4   Time|30 minutes
Nutritional Content (per serving)
Cal| 118   Fat| 7g   Protein| 10.1g   Carbs| 4.3g   Fiber| 0.8g

Ingredients:
- ❖ Eggs (6)
- ❖ Sea salt and ground black pepper, as required
- ❖ Green bell pepper (½ cup, seeded and chopped)
- ❖ Fresh chives (½ teaspoon, minced)
- ❖ Low-fat milk (½ cup)
- ❖ Fresh baby spinach (2 cups, chopped)
- ❖ Scallion (1, chopped)
- ❖ Fresh parsley (1½ tablespoons, chopped)

Directions:
1. Preheat your oven to 400 degrees F. Lightly grease a pie dish.
2. In a bowl, add eggs, milk, salt and black pepper and beat until well combined. Set aside.
3. In another bowl, add the vegetables and herbs and mix well.
4. In the bottom of prepared pie dish, place the veggie mixture evenly and top with the egg mixture.
5. Bake for approximately 20 minutes or until a wooden skewer inserted in the center comes out clean.
6. Remove pie dish from the oven and set aside for about 5 minutes before slicing.
7. Cut into desired sized wedges and serve warm.

Vanilla Waffles

Servings|2   Time|20 minutes
Nutritional Content (per serving):
Cal| 102   Fat| 0.8g   Protein| 12.1g   Carbs| 11.2g   Fiber| 0.7g

Ingredients:
- Coconut flour (¼ cup)
- Egg whites (6)
- Pure maple syrup (1 tablespoon)
- Baking powder (1 teaspoon)
- Low-fat milk (¼ cup)
- Vanilla extract (¼ teaspoon)

Directions:
1. Preheat the waffle iron and lightly grease it.
2. In a large bowl, add the flour and baking powder and mix well.
3. Add the remaining ingredients and mix until well combined.
4. Place half of the mixture in the preheated waffle iron.
5. Cook for about 3-5 minutes or until waffles become golden brown.
6. Repeat with the remaining mixture.
7. Serve warm.

Pumpkin Pancakes

Servings|10   Time|50 minutes
Nutritional Content (per serving):
Cal| 113   Fat| 4.4g   Protein| 3.6g   Carbs| 16.5g   Fiber| 2g

Ingredients:
- Eggs (2)
- Baking powder (1 tablespoon)
- Sea salt (½ teaspoon)
- Low-fat milk (¾ cup plus 2 tablespoons)
- Olive oil (2 tablespoons)
- Buckwheat flour (1 cup)
- Pumpkin pie spice (1 teaspoon)
- Pumpkin puree (1 cup)
- Pure maple syrup (3 tablespoons)
- Vanilla extract (1 teaspoon)

Directions:
1. In a blender, add all ingredients and pulse until well combined.
2. Transfer the mixture into a bowl and set aside for about 10 minutes.
3. Heat a greased non-stick skillet over medium heat.
4. Place desired amount of the mixture and spread in an even circle.
5. Cook for about 2 minutes per side.
6. Repeat with the remaining mixture.

7. Serve warm.

Chicken & Veggie Muffins

Servings|8   Time|55 minutes
Nutritional Content (per serving):
Cal| 107   Fat| 5.2g   Protein| 13.1g   Carbs| 1.7g   Fiber| 0.4g

Ingredients:
- ❖ Eggs (8)
- ❖ Filtered water (2 tablespoons)
- ❖ Cooked chicken breast (7 ounces, chopped finely)
- ❖ Fresh parsley (1 teaspoon, chopped finely)
- ❖ Sea salt and ground black pepper, as required
- ❖ Fresh spinach (1½ cups, chopped)
- ❖ Green bell pepper (1 cup, seeded and chopped finely)

Directions:
1. Preheat your oven to 350 degrees F. Grease 8 cups of a muffin tin.
2. In a bowl, add eggs, salt, black pepper and water and beat until well combined.
3. Add the chicken, spinach, bell pepper and parsley and stir to combine.
4. Place the mixture into the prepared muffin cups evenly.
5. Bake for approximately 18-20 minutes or until golden brown.
6. Remove the muffin tin from oven and place onto a wire rack to cool for about 10 minutes.
7. Carefully invert the muffins onto a platter and serve warm.

Zucchini Bread

Servings|24   Time|1 hour
Nutritional Content (per serving):
Cal| 220   Fat| 9.2g   Protein| 2.4g   Carbs| 28.5g   Fiber| 0.6g

Ingredients:

- All-purpose flour (3 cups)
- Ground cinnamon (1 teaspoon)
- (2 cups) Splenda
- Eggs (3, beaten)
- Vanilla extract (2 teaspoons)
- Baking soda (2 teaspoons)
- Ground nutmeg (1 teaspoon)
- Olive oil (1 cup)
- Zucchinis (2 cups, peeled, seeded and grated)

Directions:

1. Preheat your oven to 325 degrees F. Arrange a rack in the center of oven. Grease 2 loaf pans.
2. In a medium bowl, mix together the flour, baking soda and spices.
3. In another large bowl, add the Splenda and oil and beat until well combined.
4. Add the eggs and vanilla extract and beat until well combined.
5. Add the flour mixture and mix until just combined. Gently, fold in the zucchini.
6. Place the mixture into the bread loaf pans evenly.
7. Bake for approximately 45-50 minutes or until a toothpick inserted in the center of bread comes out clean.
8. Remove the bread pans from oven and place onto a wire rack to cool for about 15 minutes.
9. Carefully, invert the breads onto the wire rack to cool completely before slicing.
10. Cut each bread loaf into desired-sized slices and serve.

Lunch Recipes

Cucumber & Yogurt Salad

Servings|4   Time|10 minutes
Nutritional Content (per serving):
Cal| 71   Fat| 0.8g   Protein| 4g   Carbs| 13.8g   Fiber| 1.7g

Ingredients:

- ❖ Small cucumbers (4, peeled, seeded and chopped)
- ❖ Sea salt and ground black pepper, as required
- ❖ Low-fat plain Greek yogurt (½ cup)
- ❖ Fresh dill (1 teaspoon, chopped)
- ❖ Fresh lemon juice (1 tablespoon)

Directions:

1. In a salad bowl, add all the ingredients and mix well.
2. Serve immediately.

Cucumber & Tomato Salad

Servings|5   Time|10 minutes
Nutritional Content (per serving):
Cal| 68   Fat| 5.8g   Protein| 0.9g   Carbs| 4.4g   Fiber| 1.1g

Ingredients:

- ❖ Cucumbers (2 cups, peeled, seeded and chopped)
- ❖ Extra-virgin olive oil (2 tablespoons)
- ❖ Tomatoes (2 cups, peeled, seeded and chopped)
- ❖ Fresh lime juice (2 tablespoons)
- ❖ Sea salt, as required

Directions:

1. In a salad bowl, add all the ingredients and toss to coat well.
2. Serve immediately.

Beet Soup

Servings|4   Time|15 minutes
Nutritional Content (per serving):
Cal| 149   Fat| 0.6g   Protein| 11.8g   Carbs| 25.2g   Fiber| 2.5g

Ingredients:
- Fat-free plain yogurt (2 cups)
- Beets (2 cups, trimmed, peeled and chopped)
- Fresh chives (1 tablespoon, minced)
- Fresh lemon juice (1½ tablespoons)
- Fresh dill (1 teaspoon)
- Sea salt, as required

Directions:
1. In a high-powered blender, add all ingredients except for chives and pulse until smooth.
2. Transfer the soup into a pan over medium heat and cook for about 3-5 minutes or until heated through.
3. Serve immediately with the garnishing of chives.

Braised Asparagus

Servings|2   Time|18 minutes
Nutritional Content (per serving):
Cal| 82   Fat| 7.1g   Protein| 3.7g   Carbs| 2.6g   Fiber| 1.4g

Ingredients:
- Chicken bone broth (½ cup)
- Asparagus (1 cup, trimmed)
- Olive oil (1 tablespoon)
- Lemon peel (½-inch piece)

Directions:
1. In a Small pan add the broth, oil and lemon peel over medium heat and bring to a boil.
2. Add the asparagus and cook, covered for about 3-4 minutes.
3. Discard the lemon peel and serve.

Glazed Carrots

Servings|6   Time|30 minutes
Nutritional Content (per serving):
Cal| 90   Fat| 4.7g   Protein| 1g   Carbs| 12g   Fiber| 2.8g

Ingredients:

- ❖ Carrots (1½ pounds, peeled and cut into ½-inch pieces diagonally)
- ❖ Fresh orange juice (3 tablespoons)
- ❖ Filtered water (½ cup)
- ❖ Olive oil (2 tablespoons)
- ❖ Sea salt, as required

Directions:

1. In a large skillet, add the carrots, water, boil and salt over medium heat and bring to a boil.
2. Now adjust the heat to low and simmer; covered for about 6 minutes.
3. Add the orange juice and stir to combine.
4. Now adjust the heat to high and cook, uncovered for about 5-8 minutes, tossing frequently.
5. Serve immediately.

Mushroom Curry

Servings|6   Time|35 minutes
Nutritional Content (per serving):
Cal| 70   Fat| 5g   Protein| 3g   Carbs| 5.3g   Fiber| 1.4g

Ingredients:

- Tomatoes (2 cups, peeled, seeded and chopped)
- Fresh ginger (1½ tablespoons, chopped)
- Fresh shiitake mushrooms (2 cups, sliced)
- Sea salt and ground black pepper, as required
- Filtered water (1½ cups)
- Olive oil (2 tablespoons)
- Ground turmeric (¼ teaspoon)
- Fresh button mushrooms (5 cups, sliced)
- Fat-free yogurt (¼ cup, whipped)

Directions:

1. In a food processor, add the tomatoes and ¼ cup of water and pulse until a smooth paste forms.
2. In a pan, heat the oil over medium heat and sauté the ginger and turmeric for about 1 minute.
3. Add the tomato paste and cook for about 5 minutes.
4. Stir in the mushrooms, yogurt and remaining water and bring to a boil.
5. Cook for about 10-12 minutes, stirring occasionally.
6. Season with the salt and black pepper and remove from the heat.
7. Serve hot.

Squash Mac 'n Cheese

Servings|6   Time|27 minutes
Nutritional Content (per serving):
Cal| 321   Fat| 11.9g   Protein| 14g   Carbs| 40g   Fiber| 2.4g

Ingredients:
- Whole-wheat elbow macaroni (2 cups)
- Low-fat Swiss cheese (1 cup, shredded)
- Olive oil (1 tablespoon)
- Butternut squash (1½-2 cups, peeled and cubed)
- Low-fat milk (1/3 cup)
- Sea salt and ground black pepper, as required

Directions:
1. In a large pan of the salted boiling water, cook the macaroni for about 8-10 minutes.
2. Drain the macaroni and transfer into a bowl.
3. Meanwhile, in a pan of the boiling water, cook the squash cubes for about 6 minutes or until soft.
4. Drain the squash cubes completely and return to the same pan.
5. With a masher, mash the squash and place over low heat.
6. Add the cheese and milk and cook for about 2-3 minutes, stirring continuously.
7. Add the macaroni, oil, salt and black pepper and stir to combine.
8. Remove from the heat and serve hot.

Pasta with Asparagus

Servings|4   Time|20minutes
Nutritional Content (per serving):
Cal| 157   Fat| 8.4g   Protein| 8.9g   Carbs| 35.2g   Fiber| 2.4g

Ingredients:
- Olive oil (2 tablespoons)
- Sea salt and ground black pepper, as required
- Cooked hot pasta (½ pound, drained)
- Asparagus (1 pound, trimmed and cut into 1½-inch pieces)

Directions:
1. In a large cast-iron skillet, heat the oil over medium heat and cook the asparagus, salt and black pepper for about 8-10 minutes, stirring occasionally.
2. Place the hot pasta and toss to coat well.
3. Serve immediately.

Chicken & Carrot Wraps

Servings|5 Time|25 minutes
Nutritional Content (per serving):
Cal| 280   Fat| 14g   Protein| 33.2g   Carbs| 3.8g   Fiber| 0.9g

Ingredients:

For Chicken:
- ❖ Olive oil (2 tablespoons)
- ❖ Fresh ginger (1½ tablespoons, minced)
- ❖ Ground chicken (1¼ pounds)
- ❖ Sea salt and ground black pepper, as required

For Wraps:
- ❖ Romaine lettuce leaves (10)
- ❖ Carrot (1½ cups, peeled and julienned)
- ❖ Fresh parsley (1 teaspoon, chopped)
- ❖ Fresh lime juice (2 tablespoons)

Directions:
1. In a skillet, heat the oil over medium heat and sauté the ginger for about 1 minute.
2. Add the Ground chicken, salt, and black pepper and cook for about 7-9 minutes, breaking up the meat into smaller pieces with a wooden spoon.
3. Remove from the heat and set aside to cool.
4. Arrange the lettuce leaves onto serving plates.
5. Place the cooked chicken over each lettuce leaf and top with carrot and parsley.
6. Drizzle with lime juice and serve immediately.

Tuna Stuffed Avocado

Servings|2   Time|10 minutes
Nutritional Content (per serving):
Cal| 215   Fat| 11.8g   Protein| 20.6g   Carbs|7g   Fiber| 3.2g

Ingredients:

- Large avocado (1, halved and pitted)
- Fat-free yogurt (3 tablespoons)
- Fresh parsley (1 teaspoon, chopped finely)
- Water-packed tuna (1 (5-ounce) can, drained and flaked)
- Fresh lemon juice (2 tablespoons)
- Sea salt and ground black pepper, as required

Directions:

1. Carefully, remove a little flesh from each avocado half.
2. Arrange the avocado halves onto a platter and drizzle each with 1 teaspoon of lemon juice.
3. Chop the avocado flesh and transfer into a bowl.
4. In the bowl of avocado flesh, add tuna, yogurt, parsley, remaining lemon juice, salt, and black pepper, and stir to combine.
5. Divide the tuna mixture in both avocado halves evenly.
6. Serve immediately.

Chicken Kabobs

Servings|4   Time|17 minutes
Nutritional Content (per serving):
Cal| 270   Fat| 15g   Protein| 31.5g   Carbs| 0.3g   Fiber| 0.1g

Ingredients:

- Low-fat Parmesan cheese (¼ cup, grated)
- Boneless, skinless chicken breast (1¼ pounds, cut 1-inch cubes)
- (3 tablespoons) olive oil
- Fresh basil leaves (1 cup, chopped)
- Sea salt and ground black pepper, as required

Directions:

1. In a food processor, add the cheese, oil, garlic, basil, salt, and black pepper, and pulse until smooth.
2. Transfer the basil mixture into a large bowl.
3. Add the chicken cubes and mix well.
4. Cover the bowl and refrigerate to marinate for at least 4-5 hours.
5. Preheat the grill to medium-high heat. Generously, grease the grill grate.
6. Thread the chicken cubes onto pre-soaked wooden skewers.
7. Place the skewers onto the grill and cook for about 3-4 minutes.
8. Flip and cook for about 2-3 minutes more.
9. Remove from the grill and place onto a platter for about 5 minutes before serving.
10. Serve hot.

Shrimp Kabobs

Servings|4 Time|23 minutes
Nutritional Content (per serving):
Cal| 250   Fat| 14.6g   Protein| 25.9g   Carbs| 3.4g   Fiber| 0.1g

Ingredients:

- ❖ olive oil (¼ cup)
- ❖ Ground cumin (¼ teaspoon)
- ❖ Fresh lime juice (2 tablespoons)
- ❖ Sea salt and ground black pepper, as required
- ❖ Honey (1 teaspoon)
- ❖ Medium shrimp, peeled and deveined (1 pound)
- Paprika (½ teaspoon)

Directions:

1. In a large bowl, add all the ingredients except for shrimp and mix well.
2. Add the shrimp and coat with the herb mixture generously.
3. Refrigerate to marinate for at least 30 minutes.
4. Preheat the grill to medium-high heat. Grease the grill grate.
5. Thread the shrimp onto pre-soaked wooden skewers.
6. Place the skewers onto the grill and cook for about 2-4 minutes per side.
7. Remove from the grill and place onto a platter for about 5 minutes before serving.

Carrot & Turkey Soup

Servings|4 Time|55 minutes
Nutritional Content (per serving):
Cal| 436   Fat| 12g   Protein| 59g   Carbs| 20g   Fiber| 6g

Ingredients:
- Ground turkey (1/2 pound, lean)
- frozen carrot (1/2 bag)
- green peas (1/4 cup)
- chicken broth (1 can (32 ounces)
- tomatoes (2 Medium, seeded, and roughly chopped)
- garlic powder (1 teaspoon)
- paprika (1 teaspoon)
- oregano (1 teaspoon)
- bay leaf (1)

Directions:
1. Over medium heat, brown the Ground turkey in a soup pot. Add peas, frozen carrot, paprika, tomatoes, garlic powder, bay leaf, oregano, and broth.
2. Bring pot to a boil, reduce heat, cover, and simmer for 30 minutes.

Creamy Pumpkin Soup

Servings|4-6 Time|1 hour 25 minutes
Nutritional Content (per serving):
Cal| 332   Fat| 18g   Protein| 12g   Carbs| 3.2g   Fiber| 9g

Ingredients:
- pumpkin (1, cut lengthwise, seeds removed, peeled)
- sweet potato (1, cut lengthwise, peeled)
- olive oil (2 tablespoons)
- garlic cloves (4, unpeeled)
- vegetable stock (4 cups)
- light cream (1/4 cup)
- Salt

Directions:
1. Preheat oven to 375 degrees. Cut all the side of the pumpkin, shallots and sweet potato with oil.
2. Transfer your vegetables with your garlic onto a roasting pan. Set to roast for about 40 minutes or until tender.
3. Let the vegetables cool for a time and scoop out flesh of the sweet potato and pumpkin.
4. In a soup pot, place flesh of roasted vegetables, shallots and peeled garlic. Add broth and bring to a boil.
5. Reduce heat, and let it simmer, covered for 30 minutes, stir occasionally. Let the soup cool.
6. Puree soup with a hand blender, until smooth. Add cream.
7. Season to taste and simmer until warmed through, about 5 minutes.
8. Serve in warm soup bowls.

Chicken Pea Soup

Servings|4-6   Time|1 hour 10 minutes

Nutritional Content (per serving):

Cal| 176   Fat| 5g   Protein| 15g   Carbs| 18g   Fiber| 6g

Ingredients:

- chicken breast (1 pound skinless, boneless, cubed)
- olive oil (2 tablespoons)
- garlic cloves (3, minced)
- carrots (3, grated)
- bay leaf (1)
- salt (1 teaspoon)
- poultry seasoning (1 teaspoon)
- chicken broth (8 cups)
- dried split peas (1/2 cup, washed and drained)
- green peas (1 cup)

Directions:

1. Heat up the olive oil over medium heat in a soup pot. Add chicken and cook for 5 minutes, until lightly browned.
2. Add garlic, bay leaf, carrots, salt and seasoning and cook until vegetables soften, stirring occasionally.
3. Add broth and split peas to pot and bring to a boil. Reduce heat, cover and simmer on low heat for 30-45 minutes.
4. Add green peas to the soup and heat for 5 minutes, stirring to combine all ingredients.

Shrimp & Pasta Salad

Servings|2   Time|27 minutes
Nutritional Content (per serving):
Cal| 516   Fat| 20g   Protein| 32g   Carbs| 55g   Fiber| 7g

Ingredients:

- ❖ White refined pasta (1/2 pound, shells or tubes)
- ❖ shrimp (3/4 pound Medium, peeled, deveined, and cooked)
- ❖ Fresh spinach (2 cups)
- ❖ Roma tomatoes (2 medium, seeded and chopped)
- ❖ light ranch salad dressing (1/2 cup)
- ❖ basil (4 tablespoons, chopped coarsely)
- ❖ parmesan cheese (1/4 cup, grated)

Directions:

1. Bring a salted water to boil in a pot. Cook the pasta as the package instructed. Drain the water from the pasta.
2. In a bowl, combine cooked pasta, spinach, salad dressing, tomatoes and shrimp. Refrigerate for 20 minutes.
3. Toss together with basil and cheese. Serve.

Homemade Rice Salad

Servings|6 Time|23 minutes
Nutritional Content (per serving):
Cal| 425 Fat| 6g Protein| 9g Carbs| 84g Fiber| 6g

Ingredients:

- olive oil (1 1/2 tablespoons)
- green bell peppers (2 medium, seeded, chopped, cooked)
- carrots (2 medium, diced, cooked)
- mushrooms (1 cup, sliced, cooked)
- potatoes (2 medium, peeled, cooked, cubed)
- cumin (1/2 teaspoon)
- oregano (1/2 teaspoon)
- soy sauce (1 ½ tablespoons, low sodium)
- instant white rice (3 cups, cooked, cooled)
- Fresh Italian parsley (1/4 cup, chopped)
- lemon juice (2 tablespoons)

Directions:

1. Heat the olive oil up over medium heat. Cook peppers, green beans, and carrots for about 5 minutes.
2. Add mushrooms and potatoes and continue cooking 2 - 3 minutes. Add cumin, oregano and soy sauce.
3. Transfer mixture to a large salad bowl and allow to cool to room temperature.
4. Add rice, chopped parsley and lemon juice. Mix together until combined. Serve.

Haddock Noodle Soup

Servings|2 Time|25 minutes
Nutritional Content (per serving):
Cal| 509 Fat| 6g Protein| 33g Carbs| 80g Fiber| 4g

Ingredients:
For the Fish Balls:

- ❖ whole haddock fillets (7- ounces, skinned, and finely chopped)
- ❖ squid (2- ounces, cleaned)
- ❖ Pinch of sea salt flakes
- ❖ Pinch of ground white pepper
- ❖ rice wine (1 teaspoon)
- ❖ cornstarch (1 tablespoon)
- ❖ egg white (1 Large)
- ❖ oyster sauce (1 teaspoon)
- ❖ cilantro stems (1 tablespoon finely sliced)

For the Broth:

- ❖ Fresh fish stock (1 1/2 quarts)
- ❖ vermicelli noodles (7- ounces cooked, refined white)
- ❖ pinch of sea salt flakes
- ❖ Pinch of ground white pepper
- ❖ low-sodium light soy sauce (1 tablespoon)
- ❖ toasted sesame oil (1 teaspoon)

To Serve:

- ❖ chili oil (1 teaspoon, or to taste)
- ❖ Cilantro leaves
- ❖ chives (1 tablespoon, finely chopped)

Directions:

1. Put the squid and haddock into a food processor, season with the white pepper, salt, rice wine, oyster sauce, cornstarch and egg white, and blend until it is airy and light.
2. Sprinkle the coriander stems and mix well. Use 2 tablespoons, to create an oval ball out of the fish mixture.
3. Add the fish stock in a wok and bring to a simmer.
4. Add the cooked noodles and add white pepper and sea salt. Turn the heat to medium, and gently add the fish balls to the wok.
5. Cook for 3 minutes or until the fish balls float to the surface and turn opaque white. Season with the sesame oil and light soy sauce.
6. Divide the noodles between two bowls, ladle in the stock and place six fish balls into each bowl. Drizzle with the chili oil, sprinkle over the cilantro leaves and chives, and serve immediately.

Baked Chicken Breasts

Servings|4   Time|20 minutes
Nutritional Content (per serving):
Cal| 205   Fat| 10g   Protein| 27g   Carbs| 1g   Fiber| 3g

Ingredients:

- ❖ boneless, skinless chicken breasts (4)
- ❖ Extra Virgin Olive Oil (2 tablespoons)
- ❖ kosher salt (1 teaspoon)
- ❖ black pepper (1/2 teaspoon)
- ❖ garlic powder (1/2 teaspoon)
- ❖ onion powder (1/2 teaspoon)
- ❖ chili powder (1/2 teaspoon)

Directions:

1. Turn your oven on and allow to preheat up to 450 degrees F. Lightly grease a 9x13-inch baking dish.
2. Pound the chicken breasts until they are an even ¾-inch thick. Lightly coat the chicken with olive oil.
3. Whisk together the salt, pepper, garlic powder, onion powder and chili powder.
4. Season the chicken on both sides with the spice mixture and place in the prepared pan.
5. Set to bake in the preheated oven for about 20 minutes (checking after the 15-minute mark), or until the chicken is cooked through.
6. Rest for 5-10 minutes, covered with foil, then slice and serve.

Dump Pot Chicken & Rice

Servings|4   Time|35 minutes
Nutritional Content (per serving):
Cal| 177   Fat| 1g   Protein| 11g   Carbs| 31g   Fiber| 1g

Ingredients:

- chicken white meat (1 pound, strips)
- 2 cups cooked basmati rice
- water (1/4 cup)
- soy sauce (1/4 cup, low sodium)
- lemon juice (1/2 cup)
- extra-virgin olive oil (3 tablespoons)
- salt (½ teaspoon)
- Ground pepper (¼ teaspoon)
- Chives (2 tablespoons, finely chopped)

Directions:

1. Combine the water, soy sauce and lemon in a Small bowl. Mix well.
2. Heat 2 tablespoons olive oil and cook the chicken over Medium high heat in a skillet until cooked through.
3. Add the soy mixture. Simmer for 15 minutes to reduce the sauce. Add in the remaining ingredients, except chives, and season to taste.
4. Continue to cook for 4-5 minutes, or until the rice is heated through. Garnish with chives and serve.

Italian Inspired Chicken Skillet

Servings|4   Time|30 minutes
Nutritional Content (per serving):
Cal| 278   Fat| 11g   Protein| 34g   Carbs| 12g   Fiber| 8g

Ingredients:

- chicken breasts (4 large, boneless skinless cut 1/4-inch thin)
- dried oregano (1 tablespoon, divided)
- salt (1 teaspoon)
- black pepper (1 teaspoon, divided)
- olive oil (3 tablespoons)
- baby Bella mushrooms (8 ounces, cleaned, trimmed, and sliced)
- grape tomatoes (14 ounces, halved)
- garlic (2 tablespoons, Fresh, chopped)
- chicken or vegetable stock (1/2 cup)
- lemon juice (1 tablespoon, freshly squeezed)
- chicken broth (3/4 cup)
- Handful baby spinach (optional)

Directions:

1. Season the chicken on both sides with half of the oregano, salt and pepper.
2. Heat 2 tablespoons of oil in a heavy skillet and brown the chicken on both sides for 3 minutes.
3. Remove the chicken and set aside. Sauté the mushrooms in the same skillet, add another tablespoon of oil if needed.
4. Add the tomatoes, garlic and remaining oregano, salt and pepper.
5. Cook for another 3 minutes. Deglaze the pan with the chicken or vegetable stock and then stir in the chicken broth and lemon juice.
6. Bring the liquid to a boil and then return the chicken to the pan.
7. Reduce heat to medium and simmer for 8-10 minutes, or until the chicken is fully cooked and the liquid is reduced to desired consistency.
8. Serve with rice or quinoa, if desired.

Turkey Burgers with Cucumber Salad

Servings|4   Time|30 minutes
Nutritional Content (per serving):
Cal| 314   Fat| 0g   Protein| 26g   Carbs| 15g   Fiber| 3g

Ingredients:
Turkey burgers:
- turkey (1 pound, lean ground)
- egg (1 Large, beaten)
- oatmeal (½ cup)
- onions (1/3 cup, grated)
- parsley (1/3 cup, finely chopped)
- garlic (1 clove, minced)
- sea salt (½ teaspoon)
- black pepper (½ teaspoon)
- olive oil (1 tablespoon, extra-virgin)
- canola oil (2 teaspoons)

Cucumber salad:
- cucumber (1, diced small)
- chives (1/2 cup, chopped)
- ripe tomato (1 medium, finely diced)
- Freshly squeezed lime or lemon juice (2 tablespoons)
- ¼ teaspoon kosher or sea salt

Directions:
1. Combine the turkey burger ingredients, except oil, and mix well. Form into 4 patties.
2. Lightly grease the grill and grill the patties for 5-6 minutes per side on Medium high.
3. Meanwhile, combine the cucumber salad ingredients and chill until serving.

Saltfish Salad

Servings|4   Time|30 minutes
Nutritional Content (per serving):
Cal| 613   Fat| 28g   Protein| 78g   Carbs| 9g   Fiber| 4g

Ingredients:

- salted cod (1 pound)
- yellow onion (1 Large, thinly sliced)
- tomato (1 Large, diced)
- eggs (3 hard-boiled, quartered)
- green olives (12, optional)
- olive oil (1/4 cup)
- chicken or vegetable stock (1 tablespoon)

Directions:

1. Soak the cod in cold water for 15-30 minutes. Drain and place in a large pot. Cover the cod with water and bring to a boil.
2. Change the water and bring to a simmer another 3-4 times, or until the cod is reduced to the appropriate saltiness.
3. Drain and break the cod into pieces. Sauté the onion with olive oil for 5-6 minutes, or until soft.
4. Add all your ingredients to a bowl then mix until it is fully combined. Serve with rice and drizzled with olive oil.

Taco Salad

Servings|6   Time|25 minutes
Nutritional Content (per serving):
Cal| 196   Fat| 0g   Protein| 15g   Carbs| 9g   Fiber| 2g

Ingredients:
Salad:
- Ground turkey (1/2 pound)
- chili powder (1 teaspoon)
- cumin (1/2 teaspoon)
- garlic powder (1/4 teaspoon)
- sea salt (1/4 teaspoon)
- cheddar cheese, reduced fat (1/2 cup, shredded)
- romaine lettuce (3 cups, chopped)
- cherry tomatoes (1 cup, halved)
- salsa (1/2 cup)

Creamy Salsa Dressing (optional):
- Greek yogurt (2 tablespoons, plain)
- Juice of 1 lime
- salsa (1/4 cup)

Directions:
1. Brown the turkey in a skillet over Medium high heat until cooked through. Add the spices and mix well.
2. Allow the meat to cool before layering the salad. Place the salsa in the bottom of a jar or bow and top with the turkey, tomatoes, lettuce and cheese.
3. Combine the dressing ingredients in a blender or bowl and mix well. Drizzle on the dressing before serving.

Baked Sweet Potatoes

Servings|6-8   Time|40 minutes
Nutritional Content (per serving):
Cal| 790   Fat| 1g   Protein| 4g   Carbs| 20g   Fiber| 6g

Ingredients:

- sweet potatoes (4 pounds, peeled and cut to large bite-sized pieces)
- orange juice (2 cups)
- light corn syrup (3 cups)
- Ground cinnamon (1 teaspoon)
- Ground nutmeg (1 teaspoon)
- vanilla extract (¼ cup)
- lemon zest (2 teaspoons)
- flour (2 tablespoons, refined white)
- light brown sugar (1 ½ cups, packed)
- granulated sugar (1 ½ cups)

Directions:

1. Preheat oven to 350 degrees. Boil sweet potatoes until slightly underdone.
2. Drain, cool and set aside. In a large bowl, whisk together the zest, vanilla, cinnamon, nutmeg, corn syrup and orange juice.
3. In another bowl, combine sugars and both flour together. Add in your sweet potatoes to a baking dish. Top with your dry ingredient mixture then stir until coated. Pour the liquid over yams and bake for about 25 minutes.
4. Serve and enjoy!

Dinner Recipes

Salmon Salad

Servings|2   Time|15 minutes
Nutritional Content (per serving):
Cal| 131   Fat| 6g   Protein| 18g   Carbs| 1.9g   Fiber| 0.5g

Ingredients:

- Part-skim Mozzarella cheese (¼ cup, cubed)
- Fresh dill (½ teaspoon, chopped)
- Cooked salmon (6 ounces, chopped)
- Tomato (¼ cup, peeled, seeded and chopped)
- Fresh lemon juice (1 teaspoon)
- Sea salt, as required

Directions:
1. In a salad bowl, add all the ingredients and stir to combine.
2. Serve immediately.

Tuna Salad

Servings|4   Time|15 minutes
Nutritional Content (per serving):
Cal| 277   Fat| 14.5g   Protein| 31.2g   Carbs| 5.9g   Fiber| 1.1g

Ingredients:
For Dressing:

- Fresh dill (½ teaspoon, minced)
- Fresh thyme (½ teaspoon, minced)
- Olive oil (2 tablespoons)
- Fresh lime juice (1 tablespoon)
- Pinch of ground cumin
- Sea salt and ground black pepper, as required

For Salad:

- Water-packed tuna (2 (6-ounce) cans, drained and flaked)
- Hard-boiled eggs (6, sliced)
- Tomato (1 cup, peeled, seeded and chopped)
- Large cucumber (1, peeled, seeded and sliced)

Directions:
1. For dressing: in a Small bowl, add all the ingredients and beat until well combined.
2. For salad: in a salad bowl, add all the ingredients and mix well.
3. Divide the tuna mixture onto serving plates.
4. Drizzle with dressing and serve.

Shrimp Salad

Servings|5   Time|18 minutes
Nutritional Content (per serving):
Cal| 178   Fat| 8g   Protein| 21.4g   Carbs| 5g   Fiber| 1.2g

Ingredients:

- ❖ Shrimp (1 pound, peeled and deveined)
- ❖ Sea salt and ground black pepper, as required
- ❖ Fresh cilantro (1½ tablespoons, chopped finely)
- ❖ Lemon (1, quartered)
- ❖ Olive oil (2 tablespoons)
- ❖ Fresh lemon juice (2 teaspoons)
- ❖ Tomatoes (3, peeled, seeded and sliced)
- ❖ Olives (¼ cup, pitted)

Directions:

1. In a pan of the lightly salted water, add the quartered lemon and bring to a boil.
2. Add the shrimp and cook for about 2-3 minutes or until pink and opaque.
3. With a slotted spoon, transfer the shrimp into a bowl of ice water to stop the cooking process.
4. Drain the shrimp completely and then pat dry with paper towels.
5. In a Small bowl, add the oil, lemon juice, salt, and black pepper, and beat until well combined.
6. Divide the shrimp, tomato, olives, and cilantro onto serving plates.
7. Drizzle with oil mixture and serve.

Pasta Soup

Servings|5   Time|35 minutes
Nutritional Content (per serving):
Cal| 149   Fat| 0.6g   Protein| 13.6g   Carbs| 23.3g   Fiber| 3g

Ingredients:
- Potato (1, peeled and chopped)
- Chicken bone broth (5¼ cups)
- Asparagus tips (¾ pound)
- Cooked small pasta (½ cup)
- Carrot (1, peeled and chopped)
- Tomato (½ cup, peeled, seeded and chopped)
- Sea salt and ground black pepper, as required

Directions:
1. In a pan, add the potato, carrot and broth over medium-high heat and bring to a boil.
2. Now adjust the heat to low and cook, covered for about 15 minutes or until vegetables become tender.
3. Add the tomatoes and asparagus and cook or about 4-5 minutes.
4. Stir in the cooked pasta, salt and black pepper and cook for about 2-3 minutes.
5. Serve hot.

Chicken Soup

Servings|4   Time|30 minutes
Nutritional Content (per serving):
Cal| 269   Fat| 8.7g   Protein| 34.6g   Carbs| 11.9g   Fiber| 0.6g

Ingredients:
- chicken bone broth (6 cups)
- Cooked chicken breast (1½ cups, shredded)
- Fresh lemon juice (¼ cup)
- Orzo (1/3 cup)
- Large egg yolks (6)
- Sea salt and ground black pepper, as required

Directions:
1. In a large pan, add the broth over medium-high heat and bring to a boil.
2. Add the pasta and cook for about 8-9 minutes.
3. In a slowly, add in 1 cup of the hot broth, beating continuously.
4. Add the egg mixture to the pan, stirring continuously.
5. Now adjust the heat to medium and cook for about 5-7 minutes, stirring, frequently.
6. Stir in the cooked chicken, salt and black pepper and cook for about 1-2 minutes.
7. Remove from the heat and serve hot.

Seafood Stew

Servings|8 Time|32 minutes
Nutritional Content (per serving):
Cal| 173   Fat| 5.5g   Protein| 27.1g   Carbs| 3.2g   Fiber| 0.7g

Ingredients:

- ❖ Tomatoes (2½ cups, peeled, seeded and chopped)
- ❖ Shrimp (1 pound, peeled and deveined)
- ❖ Fresh parsley (1 teaspoon, chopped)
- ❖ Fish bone broth (4½ cups)
- ❖ Salmon fillets (1 pound, cubed)
- ❖ (2 tablespoons) Fresh lime juice
- ❖ Sea salt and ground black pepper, as required

Directions:

1. In a large soup pan, add the tomatoes and broth and bring to a boil.
2. Now adjust the heat to medium and simmer for about 5 minutes.
3. Add the salmon and simmer for about 3-4 minutes.
4. Stir in the shrimp and cook for about 4-5 minutes.
5. Stir in lemon juice, salt, and black pepper, and remove from heat.
6. Serve hot with the garnishing of parsley.

Simple Chicken Breast

Servings|4   Time|26 minutes
Nutritional Content (per serving):
Cal| 254   Fat| 11.3g   Protein| 36.1g   Carbs| 0g   Fiber| 0g

Ingredients:
- ❖ Boneless, skinless chicken breast halves (4 (6-ounce))
- ❖ Olive oil (2 tablespoons)
- ❖ Sea salt and ground black pepper, as required

Directions:
1. Season each chicken breast half with salt and black pepper evenly.
2. Place chicken breast halves over a rack set in a rimmed baking sheet.
3. Refrigerate for at least 30 minutes.
4. Remove from refrigerator and pat dry with paper towels.
5. In a skillet, heat the oil over medium-low heat.
6. Place the chicken breast halves, smooth-side down, and cook for about 9-10 minutes, without moving.
7. Flip the chicken breasts and cook for about 6 minutes or until cooked through.
8. Remove from the heat and let the chicken stand in the pan for about 3 minutes.
9. Now, place the chicken breasts onto a cutting board.
10. Cut each chicken breast into slices and serve.

Chicken with Bell Peppers

Servings|6   Time|35 minutes
Nutritional Content (per serving):
Cal| 226   Fat| 12.8g   Protein| 22.9g   Carbs| 4.8g   Fiber| 0.9g

Ingredients:

- Olive oil (3 tablespoons, divided)
- Boneless, skinless chicken breasts (1 pound, sliced thinly)
- Garlic powder (¼ teaspoon)
- Sea salt and ground black pepper, as required
- Large bell peppers (3, seeded and sliced)
- Dried oregano (1 teaspoon, crushed)
- Ground cumin (¼ teaspoon)
- Chicken bone broth (¼ cup)

Directions:

1. In a skillet, heat 1 tablespoon of oil over medium-high heat and cook the bell peppers for about 4-5 minutes.
2. With a slotted spoon, transfer the peppers mixture onto a plate.
3. In the same skillet, heat the remaining over medium-high heat and cook the chicken for about 8 minutes, stirring frequently.
4. Stir in the thyme, spices, salt, black pepper, and broth, and bring to a boil.
5. Add the peppers mixture and stir to combine.
6. Now adjust the heat to medium and cook for about 3-5 minutes or until all the liquid is absorbed, stirring occasionally.
7. Serve immediately.

Chicken with Mushrooms

Servings|6 Time|33 minutes
Nutritional Content (per serving):
Cal| 200   Fat| 10.4g   Protein| 24.8g   Carbs| 1.6g   Fiber| 0.5g

Ingredients:

- ❖ Olive oil (2 tablespoons, divided)
- ❖ Sea salt and ground black pepper, as required
- ❖ Fresh ginger (1½ tablespoons, grated)
- ❖ Chicken bone broth (½ cup)
- ❖ Boneless, skinless chicken breasts (4 (4-ounce), cut into small pieces)
- ❖ Fresh mushrooms (4 cups, sliced)

Directions:

1. In a large skillet, heat 1 tablespoon of oil over medium-high heat and stir fry the chicken pieces, salt, and black pepper for about 4-5 minutes or until golden-brown.
2. With a slotted spoon, transfer the chicken pieces onto a plate.
3. In the same skillet, heat the remaining oil over medium heat and sauté the onion, ginger for about 1 minute.
4. Add the mushrooms and cook for about 6-7 minutes, stirring frequently.
5. Add the cooked chicken and broth and stir fry for about 3-5 minutes
6. Add in the salt and black pepper and remove from the heat.
7. Serve hot.

Lemony Salmon

Servings|4 Time|14 minutes
Nutritional Content (per serving):
Cal| 290 Fat| 21.5g Protein| 33.2g Carbs| 1g Fiber| 0.2g

Ingredients:
- ❖ Fresh lemon zest (½ teaspoon, grated)
- ❖ Fresh lemon juice (2 tablespoons)
- ❖ Boneless, skinless salmon fillets (4 (6-ounce))
- ❖ Extra-virgin olive oil (2 tablespoons)
- ❖ Sea salt and ground black pepper, as required

Directions:
1. Preheat the grill to medium-high heat. Grease the grill grate.
2. In a bowl, place all ingredients except for salmon fillets and mix well.
3. Add the salmon fillets and coat with garlic mixture generously.
4. Place the salmon fillets onto grill and cook for about 6-7 minutes per side.
5. Serve hot.

Prawns with Asparagus

Servings|5 Time|30 minutes
Nutritional Content (per serving):
Cal| 176 Fat| 7.3g Protein| 22.7g Carbs| 5.1g Fiber| 1.9g

Ingredients:
- ❖ Olive oil (2 tablespoons)
- ❖ Asparagus (1 pound, trimmed)
- ❖ Sea salt and ground black pepper, as required
- ❖ Fresh lemon juice (2 tablespoons)
- ❖ Prawns (1 pound, peeled and deveined)
- ❖ Fresh ginger root (1 teaspoon, minced)

Directions:
1. In a skillet, heat 1 tablespoon of oil over medium-high heat and cook the prawns with salt and black pepper for about 3-4 minutes.
2. With a slotted spoon, transfer the prawns into a bowl. Set aside.
3. In the same skillet, heat the remaining oil over medium-high heat and cook the asparagus, ginger, salt and black pepper for about 6-8 minutes, stirring frequently.
4. Stir in the prawns and cook for about 1 minute.
5. Stir in the lemon juice and remove from the heat.
6. Serve hot.

Scallops with Spinach

Servings|6   Time|28 minutes
Nutritional Content (per serving):
Cal| 168   Fat| 5.9g   Protein| 21.5g   Carbs| 7.9g   Fiber| 2.1g

Ingredients:

- ❖ Fresh sea scallops (1½ pounds, side muscles removed)
- ❖ Olive oil (2 tablespoons)
- ❖ Garlic cloves (3, sliced)
- ❖ Sea salt and ground black pepper, as required
- ❖ Onion (1 cup, chopped)

Fresh baby spinach (1 pound)

Directions:

1. Sprinkle the scallops with salt and black pepper.
2. In a large skillet, heat the oil over medium-high heat and cook the scallops for about 2 minutes per side.
3. With a slotted spoon, transfer the scallops onto a plate.
4. In the same skillet, add the onion and garlic over medium heat and sauté for about 4-5 minutes.
5. Add the spinach and cook for about 2-3 minute, stirring frequently.
6. Stir in the salt and black pepper and remove from the heat.
7. Divide spinach mixture onto serving plates and top each with scallops.
8. Serve immediately.

Garlic Parmesan Chicken & Potatoes

Servings|2 Time|50 minutes
Nutritional Content (per serving):
Cal| 382   Fat| 23g   Protein| 10g   Carbs| 24g   Fiber| 6g

Ingredients:

- chicken thighs (6 bone-in, skin-on)
- Italian seasoning (1 tablespoon)
- Salt (kosher) and Grounded black pepper, to taste
- butter (3 tablespoons, unsalted, divided)
- baby spinach (3 cups, roughly chopped)
- baby Dutch potatoes (16 ounces, halved)
- Fresh parsley leaves (2 tablespoons, chopped)

- For the garlic parmesan cream sauce
- butter (1/4 cup, unsalted)
- garlic (4 cloves, minced)
- cream cheese (2 tablespoons)
- chicken broth (1/2 cup)
- dried thyme (1 tablespoon)
- dried basil (1/2 teaspoon)
- half and half (1/2 cup)
- Parmesan (1/2 cup, Freshly grated)
- Salt (kosher) & Grounded black pepper, to taste

Directions:

1. Turn your oven on and allow to preheat up to 400 degrees F and lightly grease a 9x13-inch baking dish.
2. Season the chicken with Italian seasoning, salt and pepper. Sear the chicken for 2-3 minutes per side in 2 tablespoons of butter in a large skillet.
3. Remove and set aside. Add the remaining butter into the skillet and cook the spinach for 2 minutes, or until wilted.
4. Melt the butter in a skillet and sauté the garlic for 1-2 minutes. Melt the cream cheese and then stir in the chicken broth, thyme and basil.
5. Cook for 1-2 minutes. Stir in the half and half and cheese until thickened, about 2 minutes. Season to taste with salt and pepper.
6. Place the chicken in the baking dish and top with the potatoes, spinach and then pour the cream sauce over the top. Bake for 25-30 minutes, or until cooked through. Garnish with parsley before serving.

Turkey & Vegetable Quesadillas

Servings|4   Time|20 minutes
Nutritional Content (per serving):
Cal| 243   Fat| 9.5g   Protein| 26g   Carbs| 15g   Fiber| 2g

Ingredients:

- Greek yogurt (¼ cup, Low-fat, plain)
- Turkey breast (12 ounces boneless and skinless)
- Ranch Seasoning Blend (2 teaspoons)
- canola oil (1 teaspoon)
- orange bell peppers (2, top and bottom removed, cored and seeded)
- tortillas (4, refined white)
- tomatoes (2, diced, seedless)
- pepper Jack cheese (½ cup shredded)

Directions:

1. Create a sauce by combining a half of a teaspoon of your seasoning blend with your yogurt. Cover and set to chill.
2. Transfer your turkey to a plastic bag then pound with a meat mallet to ¼-inch thickness. Add in your remaining seasoning and oil.
3. Leave your meat to marinate for at least 10 mins. Set a skillet on moderate heat to get hot then add in your peppers.
4. Press your peppers down for about 2 minutes to sear. Cool and dice.
5. Add your turkey into your skillet and toss the marinade. Cook over medium heat for 5 minutes.
6. Flip, and continue to cook until done (should be at 165° F). Transfer to a plate, cool and dice. Clean the skillet using paper towels.
7. Replace on medium heat. Place a tortilla in your skillet, top with half of the peppers, cheese, tomatoes, and peppers.
8. Cover with a second tortilla then cook for another 2 minutes per side. Transfer to a cutting board. Use a pizza cutter to slice in half then serve.

Roasted Salmon

Servings|4   Time|25 minutes
Nutritional Content (per serving):
Cal| 222   Fat| 1g   Protein| 26g   Carbs| 4g   Fiber| 1g

Ingredients:

- Salmon (1 whole, 2 ½- pounds, cleaned and scaled)
- Garlic-Infused (3 tablespoons)
- Kosher salt
- Freshly Ground black pepper
- Fresh flat leaf parsley (¼ cup, chopped)
- Fresh herb of your choice (¼ cup, chopped)
- Scallions (¼ cup chopped, green parts only)
- lemon (1, thinly sliced crosswise)

Directions:

1. Position rack in upper third of oven. Preheat the oven to 450°F. Prepare a rimmed roasted pan for your fish.
2. Allow to stand at room temperature while your oven preheats.
3. Place fish on pan and make 3 crosswise slashes, all the way down to the bone, on each side of the fish.
4. Use your garlic oil to rub your inside and out then season to your liking. Toss your Scallions and herbs together.
5. Press some of your herbs and a lemon slice on each serving then use the remainder to stuff the fish cavity.
6. Set to roast until done (about 20 mins). Enjoy!

Chicken & Veggie Quesadillas

Servings|4   Time|20 minutes
Nutritional Content (per serving):
Cal| 243   Fat| 9g   Protein| 26g   Carbs| 15g   Fiber| 2g

Ingredients:

- Greek yogurt (¼ cup, Low-fat, plain)
- Chicken breast (12 ounces boneless and skinless)
- Ranch Seasoning Blend (2 teaspoons)
- canola oil (1 teaspoon)
- orange bell peppers (2, top and bottom removed, cored, and seeded)
- tortillas (4, refined white)
- tomatoes (2, diced, seedless)
- pepper Jack cheese (½ cup shredded)

Directions:

1. Create a sauce by combining a half of a teaspoon of your seasoning blend with your yogurt. Cover and set to chill.
2. Transfer your chicken to a plastic bag then pound with a meat mallet to ¼-inch thickness. Add in your remaining seasoning and oil.
3. Leave your meat to marinate for at least 10 mins. Set a skillet on moderate heat to get hot then add in your peppers.
4. Press your peppers down for about 2 minutes to sear. Cool and dice.
5. Add your chicken into your skillet and toss the marinade. Cook over medium heat for 5 minutes.
6. Flip, and continue to cook until done (should be at 165° F). Transfer to a plate, cool and dice. Clean the skillet using paper towels.
7. Replace on medium heat. Place a tortilla in your skillet, top with half of the peppers, cheese, tomatoes, and peppers.
8. Cover with a second tortilla then cook for another 2 minutes per side. Transfer to a cutting board.
9. Use a pizza cutter to slice in half then serve.

Fajita Stuffed Chicken

Servings|2 Time|45minutes
Nutritional Content (per serving):
Cal| 591   Fat| 18g   Protein| 60g   Carbs| 45g   Fiber| 4g

Ingredients:

- chicken breasts (4)
- olive oil (2 tablespoons)
- taco seasoning (2 tablespoons)
- ½ each red, yellow and green pepper, diced
- red onion (1 Small, diced)
- shredded cheese (1/2 cup, shredded)
- cilantro (optional for garnish)
- Salsa and sour cream

- Roasted sweet potatoes (optional side)
- olive oil (1 tablespoon)
- sweet potatoes (3, cut into 1-inch pieces)
- chili powder (2 teaspoons)
- paprika (2 teaspoons)
- garlic powder (2 teaspoons)
- salt (1 teaspoon)

Directions:

1. Turn your oven on and allow to preheat up to 450 degrees F.
2. Coat the sweet potatoes in olive oil and the spices and roast in a baking dish or sheet pan for 25-30 minutes, or until tender.
3. Meanwhile, make a slit in the side of each chicken breast. Combine the bell peppers and onions and stuff into the slit.
4. Grill the chicken for 15 minutes on Medium high. Sprinkle on the cheese and grill for another 5 minutes, or until the cheese is melted.
5. Serve with the sweet potatoes and other toppings of choice.

Chicken Chili with Winter Squash

Servings|8   Time|1 hour
Nutritional Content (per serving):
Cal| 298   Fat| 1g   Protein| 34g   Carbs| 28g   Fiber| 2g

Ingredients:

- Garlic-Infused oil (3 tablespoons)
- Ground chicken (2- pounds)
- leeks (3/4 cup finely chopped, green parts only)
- Scallions (1/4 cup (16, finely chopped, green parts only)
- green bell pepper (1, cored, finely chopped)
- red bell pepper (1, cored, finely chopped)
- cumin (1 tablespoons)
- paprika (1 teaspoon)
- smoked paprika (1 teaspoon)
- chile powder (¼ to ½ teaspoon)
- dried oregano (1/2 teaspoon)
- kosher salt (1/2 teaspoon)
- Freshly Ground black pepper (¼ teaspoon)
- Chicken Stock (2 cups)
- Tomatoes (2 (14.5 ounces) cans diced, drained well)
- Tomato Sauce (1, 15-ounce)
- butternut squash (10 ½ ounces, peeled, cut into Large bite-sized chunks)
- black beans (7- ounces, drained, canned)
- fine Ground yellow cornmeal (1/4 cup)

Directions:

1. Heat 1 tablespoon of oil in a heavy bottomed large Dutch oven over low-medium heat and add the Ground chicken, breaking it up with a spatula.
2. Sauté until the chicken loses all of its pink color. Remove from pan and set aside.
3. Add in the rest of your oil on low-Medium heat. Once hot, add in your Scallions and leeks then until tender (about 2 minutes). Add in the chopped peppers and sauté until crisp-tender.
4. Stir in the spices, salt and pepper, using smaller amount of hot chile.
5. Sauté for about 15 seconds, then add the reserved chicken. Stir in your tomatoes, tomato sauce, squash and stock.
6. Cover adjust heat and cook for about 20 to 30 minutes or until squash is tender. Taste and adjust seasoning as desired.
7. Combine your cornmeal with a ladle of the chili liquid to make a paste.
8. Stir your cornmeal paste into the chili and distribute well. Cover then allow to simmer for about another 5 minutes to thicken. Serve hot.

Grilled Lemon Rosemary Chicken

Servings|8 Time|18 minutes
Nutritional Content (per serving):
Cal| 251 Fat| 11g Protein| 35g Carbs| 1g Fiber| 3g

Ingredients:

- chicken breast fillets (2 pounds.)
- olive oil (1/4 cup)
- garlic (3 cloves, minced)
- zest from one lemon
- juice from one lemon (about ¼ cup)
- salt (3/4 teaspoon)
- pepper (1/4 teaspoon)
- rosemary (1 Large sprig)

Directions:

1. Combine all ingredients in a bag and mix well. Refrigerate for 3 hours to allow the chicken to marinate.
2. Grill over medium heat for 3-4 minutes per side, or until cooked through. Serve hot.

Spaghetti Squash in Tomato Sauce

Servings|2 Time|1 hour 10 minutes
Nutritional Content (per serving):
Cal| 113 Fat| 8g Protein| 2g Carbs| 12g Fiber| 2g

Ingredients:

- Spaghetti Squash (1 cup)
- Olive Oil (1 tablespoon)
- Seasonings, to taste
- tomato sauce (1 cup)

Directions:

1. Cut spaghetti squash in half and drizzle with olive oil. Sprinkle on desired seasonings and bake cut-side-down at 400 degrees for about an hour.
2. The squash should be very tender when finished. Allow squash to cool for a few minutes, then take a fork and scrape out the squash "noodles".
3. Serve and cover with lemon juice, olive oil, and garlic or the spaghetti sauce of your choosing.

Jalapeño Turkey Burgers

Servings|4   Time|20 minutes
Nutritional Content (per serving):
Cal| 248   Fat| 9g   Protein| 25g   Carbs| 19g   Fiber| 1g

Ingredients:

- Ground turkey (1 pound)
- jalapeño pepper, (3/4, minced)
- shallot (1 med., peeled and minced)
- Lime (1, zested with 2 teaspoons juice)
- cilantro (2 tablespoons, chopped)
- paprika (1 teaspoon)
- cumin (1 teaspoon)
- sea salt (1/2 teaspoon)
- black pepper (1/2 teaspoon)
- guacamole
- Pico de Gallo

Directions:

1. Add all your ingredients to a bowl then mix until it is fully combined. Form to make 4 patties.
2. Preheat a skillet with a little olive oil in it on Medium heat. Cook the patties for 5 minutes per side, or until cooked through.
3. Serve with guacamole, Pico de Gallo or toppings of choice.

Crock Pot Thai Turkey Curry

Servings|2   Time|14 minutes
Nutritional Content (per serving):
Cal| 436   Fat| 28g   Protein| 28g   Carbs| 24g   Fiber| 3g

Ingredients:

- water (2 cups)
- Thai red curry paste (2-4 tablespoons, or to taste)
- soy sauce (1 tablespoon)
- minced ginger (1 tablespoon)
- fish sauce (2 teaspoons)
- garlic cloves (3, minced)
- turkey thighs (1 pound boneless, skinless, cut into 2-3 pieces
- Kabocha squash (1 Large, cut into 1 – inch cubes)
- yellow onion (1 Medium, chopped)
- chili peppers (1-2, optional)
- coconut milk (1 14 ounces can)
- Kale (1 bunch, torn)
- cilantro and lime wedges for serving

Directions:

1. Add all the ingredients, with the exception of your coconut milk and kale in a slow cooker and mix well.
2. Cook on high for 4 hours and then stir in the coconut milk and kale.
3. Mix well and cook on high for another 15-20 minutes, or until hot through and the kale has wilted.
4. Season to taste with salt and pepper and serve with cilantro and lime wedges.

Creamy Sun-dried Tomato Turkey

Servings|8 Time|1½ hours
Nutritional Content (per serving):
Cal| 162   Fat| 8g   Protein| 16g   Carbs| 7g   Fiber| 2g

Ingredients:

- Salt (1 tablespoon)
- Freshly Ground Pepper (1 teaspoon)
- Turkey thighs (8, bone-in, skin removed)
- Extra Virgin Olive Oil (3 tablespoons)
- Yellow Onion (1, sliced thinly)
- Sun-dried Tomatoes (¾ cup, sliced)
- Garlic (1 tablespoon, minced)
- Italian Seasoning (1 teaspoon)
- Large pinch Red Pepper Flakes
- Coconut Milk (13.5 ounces can)
- Turkey Stock (1 cup)
- Basil shredded, to top

Directions:

1. Turn your oven on and allow to preheat up to 400 degrees F. Thoroughly season your turkey with your salt and pepper.
2. Fry the turkey, in an oven safe skillet, in the olive oil for 2-3 minutes, or until browned on all sides. Set aside.
3. Add a little more oil to the pan and sauté the onion for 2 minutes. Add the Italian seasoning, garlic, tomatoes and red pepper and cook for 30 seconds.
4. Stir in the coconut milk and chicken broth and bring the mixture to a boil. Place the turkey back into the sauce and spoon some sauce on top.
5. Cover and bake for 45 minutes. Reduce heat to 300 degrees F and cook for another 20 minutes. Garnish with basil before serving.

White Mushroom & Carrot Soup

Servings|4   Time|35 minutes
Nutritional Content (per serving):
Cal| 219   Fat| 12g   Protein| 13g   Carbs| 15g   Fiber| 3g

Ingredients:

- ❖ olive oil (2 tablespoons)
- ❖ carrots (2, chopped)
- ❖ white mushrooms (5 cups, sliced)
- ❖ smoked ham (1 ½ cups, diced)
- ❖ garlic powder (2 teaspoons)
- ❖ chicken broth (2 (14 ounces) can)
- ❖ stewed tomatoes (1 (14 ounces) can, seedless)

Directions:

1. Heat the oil up over medium heat, in a soup pot. Add carrots; cook, stir often, for 5 minutes.
2. Add mushrooms; cook, stirring frequently for 5 minutes. Add ham, garlic powder, chicken broth and tomatoes.
3. Bring to a boil; reduce heat and simmer covered for 10 minutes. Serve.

Shitake & Ginger Soup

Servings|4   Time|35 minutes
Nutritional Content (per serving):
Cal| 117   Fat| 3g   Protein| 4g   Carbs| 19g   Fiber| 1g

Ingredients:

- vegetable oil (2 teaspoons)
- garlic cloves (3, crushed and peeled)
- Fresh ginger (1 tablespoon, finely shredded)
- Shitake mushrooms (4 ounces, sliced)
- vegetable stock (4 cups)
- light soy sauce (1 teaspoon, optional)
- bean sprouts (4 ounces)
- thin spaghetti pasta (4 ounces, white)
- Fresh cilantro (4 tablespoons)

Directions:

1. Bring a salted water to boil in a pot. Add the pasta and cook as the package instructed.
2. While pasta is cooking, in a large soup pot, heat oil over medium heat. Add garlic, ginger and mushrooms.
3. Stir until softened, about 3-4 minutes. Add vegetable stock and bring to boil.
4. Add soy sauce and bean sprouts and continue to cook until tender. Serve and garnish with fresh cilantro.

Phase: 3- High-Fiber Recipes

Breakfast Recipes

Apple, Grapefruit & Carrot Juice

Servings|2   Time|10 minutes
Nutritional Content (per serving):
Cal| 265   Fat| 0.7g   Protein| 4.3g   Carbs| 67g   Fiber| 11.7g

Ingredients:
- ❖ Large Granny Smith apples (2, cored and sliced
- ❖ Medium grapefruit (2, peeled and seeded)
- ❖ Medium carrots (4, peeled and chopped)
- ❖ Fresh kale (1 cup)
- ❖ Fresh lemon juice (1 teaspoon)

Directions:
1. Place all the ingredients in a blender and pulse until well combined.
2. Through a cheesecloth-lined strainer, strain the juice and transfer into 2 glasses.
3. Serve immediately.

Pear, Celery & Kale Juice

Servings|2   Time|10 minutes
Nutritional Content (per serving):
Cal| 209   Fat| 0.9g   Protein| 5.1g   Carbs| 50.5g   Fiber| 15.2g

Ingredients:
- ❖ Pears (6, cored and chopped
- ❖ Fresh kale (3 cups)
- ❖ Celery stalks (3)
- ❖ Fresh parsley (1 teaspoon)

Directions:
1. Place all the ingredients in a blender and pulse until well combined.
2. Through a cheesecloth-lined strainer, strain the juice and transfer into 2 glasses.
3. Serve immediately.

Oats & Apple Smoothie

Servings|4 Time|10 minutes
Nutritional Content (per serving):
Cal| 434   Fat| 6.4g   Protein| 38.7g   Carbs| 55.3g   Fiber| 7.1g

Ingredients:

- Rolled oats (2 ounces)
- Unsweetened vegan protein powder (4 scoops)
- Ground cinnamon (1 teaspoon)
- Milk (2 cups)
- Apples (4, peeled, cored and chopped roughly)
- Stevia powder (1 teaspoon)
- Plain yogurt (17 ounces)
- Ice cubes (6-8)

Directions:
1. In a high-speed blender, add all the ingredients and pulse until smooth and creamy.
2. Transfer the smoothie into 4 serving glasses and serve immediately.

Oats & Peach Smoothie

Servings|2 Time|10 minutes
Nutritional Content (per serving):
Cal| 328   Fat| 4.1g   Protein| 15g   Carbs| 56g   Fiber| 5g

Ingredients:

- Frozen peaches (2 cups, pitted)
- Ground cinnamon (¼ teaspoon)
- Fresh orange juice (½ cup)
- Rolled oats (½ cup)
- Plain yogurt (1½ cups)

Directions:
1. In a high-speed blender, add all the ingredients and pulse until smooth and creamy.
2. Transfer the smoothie into 2 serving glasses and serve immediately.

Spinach & Avocado Smoothie Bowl

Servings|2 Time|10 minutes
Nutritional Content (per serving):
Cal| 471 Fat| 23.5g Protein| 36.2g Carbs| 32.2g Fiber| 8g

Ingredients:
- ❖ Fresh spinach (2 cups)
- ❖ Unsweetened vegan protein powder (2 scoops)
- ❖ (2 tablespoons) Fresh lemon juice
- ❖ Ice cubes (4-6)
- ❖ Medium avocado (1, peeled, pitted and chopped roughly)
- ❖ Pure maple syrup (3 tablespoons)
- ❖ Milk (1 cup)

Directions:
1. In a high-speed blender, place all ingredients and pulse until creamy.
2. Pour into 2 serving bowls and serve immediately with your favorite topping.

Apple & Banana Porridge

Servings|4 Time|14 minutes
Nutritional Content (per serving):
Cal| 194 Fat| 3g Protein| 5.9g Carbs| 40.9g Fiber| 6g

Ingredients:
- ❖ Milk (2 cups)
- ❖ Vanilla extract (½ teaspoon)
- ❖ Pinch of ground cinnamon
- ❖ Small apple (½, cored and sliced)
- ❖ Large apples (3, peeled, cored and grated)
- ❖ Banana (1, peeled and sliced)

Directions:
1. In a large pan, add the milk, grated apples, vanilla extract and cinnamon and mix well.
2. Place the pan over medium-low heat and cook for about 3-4 minutes, stirring occasionally.
3. Transfer the porridge into the serving bowls.
4. Top with the banana and apple slices and serve.

Bulgur Porridge

Servings|2   Time|25 minutes
Nutritional Content (per serving):
Cal| 231   Fat| 2.4g   Protein| 6.5g   Carbs| 50.6g   Fiber| 8.5g

Ingredients:

- ❖ Milk (2/3 cup)
- ❖ Pinch of sea salt
- ❖ Large apple (1, peeled, cored and chopped)
- ❖ Bulgur (1/3 cup, rinsed)
- ❖ Ripe banana (1, peeled and mashed)

Directions:

1. In a pan, add the milk, bulgur and salt over medium-high heat and bring to a boil.
2. Now adjust the heat to low and simmer for about 10 minutes.
3. Remove the pan of bulgur from heat and immediately, stir in the mashed banana.
4. Serve warm with the topping of chopped apple.

Pumpkin Oatmeal

Servings|2   Time|12 minutes
Nutritional Content (per serving):
Cal| 268   Fat| 2.4g   Protein| 28.4g   Carbs| 34.4g   Fiber| 5g

Ingredients:

- ❖ Hot water (2 cups)
- ❖ rolled oats (1/3 cup)
- ❖ Ground cinnamon (1 teaspoon)
- ❖ Ground nutmeg (¼ teaspoon)
- ❖ Pure maple syrup (1 tablespoon)
- ❖ Small banana (1, peeled and sliced)
- ❖ pumpkin puree (1/3 cup)
- ❖ Ground cinnamon (1 teaspoon)
- ❖ Ground ginger (1 teaspoon)
- ❖ Unsweetened vanilla vegan protein powder (2 scoops)

Directions:

1. In a microwave-safe bowl, place water, pumpkin puree, oats, chia seeds and spices and mix well.
2. Microwave on High for about 2 minutes.
3. Remove the bowl of oatmeal from the microwave and stir in the protein powder and maple syrup.
4. Top with banana slices and serve immediately.

Oats & Quinoa Porridge

Servings|3   Time|30 minutes
Nutritional Content (per serving):
Cal| 384   Fat| 6.5g   Protein| 12.2g   Carbs| 72g   Fiber| 7g

Ingredients:

- ❖ Milk (2 cups)
- ❖ Old-fashioned oats (1 cup)
- ❖ Pure maple syrup (3 tablespoons)
- ❖ Small apple (1, peeled, cored and chopped)
- ❖ Filtered water (2 cups)
- ❖ Dried quinoa (1/3 cup, rinsed)
- ❖ Vanilla extract (½ teaspoon)
- ❖ Large banana (1, peeled and sliced)

Directions:

1. In a pan, mix together all the ingredients except for banana and apple over medium heat and bring to a gentle boil.
2. Cook for about 20 minutes, stirring occasionally.
3. Remove from the heat and serve warm with the garnishing of banana and apple.

Savory Crepes

Servings|2   Time|30 minutes
Nutritional Content (per serving):
Cal| 229   Fat| 3.8g   Protein| 12.1g   Carbs| 38.1g   Fiber| 11g

Ingredients:

- ❖ Chickpea flour (1¼ cups)
- ❖ Red chili powder (¼ teaspoon)
- ❖ Filtered water (1½ cups)
- ❖ Sea salt, as required

Directions:

1. In a blender, add all the ingredients and pulse until well combined.
2. Heat a lightly greased nonstick skillet over medium-high heat.
3. Add the desired amount of the mixture and tilt the pan to spread it evenly.
4. Cook for about 3 minutes.
5. Carefully, flip the crepe and cook for about 1-2 minutes.
6. Repeat with the remaining mixture.
7. Serve warm.

Eggless Veggie Omelet

Servings|4 Time|27 minutes
Nutritional Content (per serving):
Cal| 172   Fat| 8.8g   Protein| 6g   Carbs| 18.5g   Fiber| 3.9g

Ingredients:
- Chickpea flour (1 cup)
- Red chili powder (¼ teaspoon)
- Pinch of sea salt
- Medium onion (1, chopped finely)
- Fresh cilantro (2 tablespoons, chopped)
- olive oil (2 tablespoons, divided)
- Ground turmeric (¼ teaspoon)
- Pinch of ground cumin
- Filtered water (1½-2 cups)

Medium tomatoes (2, peeled, seeded and chopped finely)

Directions:
1. In a large bowl, add the flour, spices, and salt and mix well.
2. Slowly, add the water and mix until well combined.
3. Fold in the onion, tomatoes and cilantro.
4. In a large non-stick frying pan, heat ½ tablespoon of oil over medium heat.
5. Add ½ of the tomato mixture and tilt the pan to spread it.
6. Cook for about 5-7 minutes.
7. Place the ½ tablespoon of oil over the omelet and carefully flip it over.
8. Cook for about 4-5 minutes or until golden brown.
9. Repeat with the remaining oil and mixture.

Grilled Vegetable Sandwich

Servings|4   Time|22 minutes
Nutritional Content (per serving):
Cal| 681   Fat| 66g   Protein| 16g   Carbs| 14g   Fiber| 6g

Ingredients:

- Japanese eggplant (1, sliced in half-inch thick slices)
- Zucchini (1 Small, sliced in half-inch thick slices)
- red pepper (1, seeded and quartered)
- Portobello mushroom caps (2)
- extra-virgin olive oil (1/2 cup)
- salt (1/4 teaspoon)
- goat cheese (6 ounces)
- whole wheat (8 slices)
- baby spinach (1 cup)

Directions:

1. With a pastry brush, brush olive oil on the vegetable slices and the mushrooms caps.
2. Season them with salt. Put the vegetables on the grill and cook it until they are tender.
3. To assemble, slice the mushrooms, spread goat cheese on both sides of the bread.
4. Add the grilled vegetables of each variation and a quarter of the mushrooms.
5. Cover with spinach and top with bread before serving.

Spinach and Ham Pizza

Servings|4 Time|22 minutes
Nutritional Content (per serving):
Cal| 256   Fat| 19g   Protein| 18g   Carbs| 4g   Fiber| 1g

Ingredients:

- store-bought baked thin-crust whole wheat pizza shell (1)
- baby spinach leaves (4 cups, thinly sliced)
- olive oil (2 teaspoons)
- ham (3 ounces, thinly sliced)
- Feta cheese (1/4, crumbled)
- Parmesan cheese (1/4 cup grated)
- cloves (3, thinly sliced garlic)

Directions:
1. Preheat oven to 450 degrees F. Place the pizza shell on a cookie sheet.
2. Scatter spinach all over crust. Drizzle with oil. Place ham, garlic, and cheeses on top of spinach.
3. Bake for 10-12 minutes, until spinach is wilted.

Fruit Bowl

Servings|4 Time|5 minutes
Nutritional Content (per serving):
Cal| 308   Fat| 1g   Protein| 4g   Carbs| 79g   Fiber| 13g

Ingredients:

- Pears (1 cup, cut in half-inch cubes)
- Bananas (1 cup, cut in half-inch cubes)
- Oranges (1 cup, cut in half-inch cubes)

Directions:
1. Mix all ingredients together and serve with a salad dressing.

Easy Tofu & Beans

Servings|4   Time|35 minutes
Nutritional Content (per serving):
Cal| 678   Fat| 44g   Protein| 19g   Carbs| 55g   Fiber| 6g

Ingredients:

- firm tofu (1 (14 ounces) pkg., drained, cut in cubes)
- whole wheat flour (1/4 cup)
- canola oil (1 tablespoon)
- olive oil (1/2 cup)
- balsamic vinegar (2 tablespoons)
- Dijon mustard (1 tablespoon)
- soy sauce (3 tablespoons)
- onions (1/2 cup, sliced)
- carrots (1/2 cups, sliced)
- green beans (1 cup, ends cut)
- Fresh soybeans (1/2 cups)
- cabbage (1 1/2 cups, chopped)
- brown rice (1 cup, cooked)

Directions:

1. In a shallow bowl or plate, mix tofu with flour until evenly coated. Heat up the canola oil over medium heat, in a non-stick pan.
2. Add tofu and cook until lightly brown. Remove from pan and put aside.
3. Prepare dressing by whisking together olive oil, vinegar, mustard and soy sauce.
4. In same pan, combine 2 tablespoons of the dressing mixture with onions, carrots, green beans, soybeans and cabbage.
5. Stir fry for 10 minutes. Add remaining dressing mixture and tofu. Mix. Cook for 2 minutes, stirring gently.
6. Serve over hot brown rice.

Couscous with Dates

Servings|4   Time|20 minutes
Nutritional Content (per serving):
Cal| 197   Fat| 4g   Protein| 6g   Carbs| 33g   Fiber| 2g

Ingredients:

- Water (1/2 cup)
- turkey stock (1 cup)
- olive oil (1 tablespoon)
- dried dates (1/2 cup, chopped)
- couscous (1 cup)

- spinach (1 cup, chopped)
- lemon juice (1/2 teaspoon)
- salt (1/2 teaspoon)

Directions:

1. In a medium saucepan, over high heat, bring water, chicken broth, oil and dates to a boil. Remove from heat and stir in couscous.
2. Cover and let sit for 5-10 minutes. Stir in spinach into couscous. Add lemon juice and salt and fluff together with a fork. Serve.

Pork Fajitas

Servings|4   Time|25 minutes
Nutritional Content (per serving):
Cal| 286   Fat| 13g   Protein| 32g   Carbs| 10g   Fiber| 2g

Ingredients:

- flank steak (5 ounces, trimmed of excess fat)
- lime juice (2 teaspoons)
- garlic (1 teaspoon, chopped)
- extra virgin olive oil (1 teaspoon, divided)
- can red beans (1 (15 ounces), drained and rinsed)
- green bell pepper (1/2 cup, thinly sliced)
- red bell pepper (1/2 cup, thinly sliced)
- Scallions (1 tablespoon, chopped finely)
- Salt to taste
- whole wheat tortillas (4)

Directions:

1. Season flank steak with salt. Let sit for 10 minutes. Put the flank steak on the grill over high heat until cooked on both sides.
2. Transfer to a new plate to rest (about 10 minutes). Slice steak against the grain.
3. In a small bowl, whisk together lime juice, garlic, and olive oil. Set aside.
4. In a separate bowl, combine beans, bell peppers and scallions and season with salt. To assemble, place your steak inside your tortillas.
5. Add your bean mixture on top then sprinkle with lime sauce. Roll into fajita and serve immediately.

Cottage Crunch Wraps

Servings|2 Time|10 minutes
Nutritional Content (per serving):
Cal| 194 Fat| 3g Protein| 19g Carbs| 24g Fiber| 4g

Ingredients:

- cottage cheese (3/4 cup)
- carrots (1/4 cup, grated)
- Scallions (1/4 cup, sliced finely)
- tomatoes (1/2 cup, seeded and chopped)
- cabbage (1/2 cup, chopped)
- lime juice (1 teaspoon)
- whole wheat tortillas (2 round)

Directions:

1. In a bowl, place cheese, carrots, onions, cabbage, and tomatoes and mix well.
2. Add lime juice. Place mixture in tortillas, wrap and serve.

Bean & Vegetable Pasta

Servings|4   Time|36 minutes
Nutritional Content (per serving):
Cal| 232   Fat| 16g   Protein| 17g   Carbs| 17g   Fiber| 3g

Ingredients:

- whole wheat penne pasta (1 pound)
- olive oil (2 tablespoons)
- cloves garlic (2, minced)
- tomatoes (3 cups, seeded and chopped)
- cannellini beans (1 (14 ounces) can, drained and rinsed)
- tomato sauce (1 cup)
- spinach (2 cups, washed and chopped)
- crumbled feta cheese (1/2 cup)

Directions:

1. Bring a salted water to boil in a pot. Add the pasta then ensure to follow the cooking instructions on the package. Then drain it.
2. Set your oil to get hot on Medium heat in a nonstick pan. Cook garlic for 3 - 4 minutes. Add tomatoes, beans and tomato sauce.
3. Bring to a boil. Reduce the heat, cover and let simmer for 10 minutes. Add spinach to the sauce and let simmer for another 5 minutes or until spinach wilts.
4. Transfer to a large bowl. Combine with your sauce the top with feta. Toss to combine. Serve.

Vegetarian Penne Pasta

Servings|2   Time|26 minutes
Nutritional Content (per serving):
Cal| 283   Fat| 17g   Protein| 10g   Carbs| 32.8g   Fiber| 4g

Ingredients:

- whole wheat penne (1/2 pound)
- salt (1 tablespoon)
- extra virgin olive oil (2 tablespoons)
- white mushrooms (8 ounces sliced)
- asparagus (8 ounces, chopped thawed)
- red bell pepper (8 ounces, seeded and chopped)
- Parmesan cheese (1/4 cup, grated)
- Fresh basil (1/4 cup, chopped)

Directions:

1. Bring a salted water to boil in a pot. Add pasta and cook until it is al dente or follow the instructions on the package.
2. While the pasta is cooking, in a medium pan, heat olive oil over medium heat. Add the mushrooms and cook for five minutes.
3. Add the bell pepper and asparagus. Sauté for 4 minutes. Add the cooked pasta in the pan and add cheese, stir until well combined.
4. Put the mixture in a serving bowl, garnish with basil and serve.

Black Bean Pita Pockets

Servings|4   Time|20 minutes
Nutritional Content (per serving):
Cal| 54   Fat| 1g   Protein| 11g   Carbs| 3g   Fiber| 4g

Ingredients:

- ❖ Black beans (1 (15 ounces) can, rinsed and drained)
- ❖ artichoke hearts (1 (6 ounces) can, marinated, quartered, liquid reserved)
- ❖ black olives (1 tablespoon, sliced)
- ❖ green olives (1 tablespoon, sliced)
- ❖ green bell pepper (1 Small, seeded and diced)
- ❖ red bell pepper (1 Small, seeded and diced)
- ❖ red onion (1 Small, thinly sliced)
- ❖ red wine vinegar (2 tablespoons)
- ❖ basil (1/2 cup, chopped)
- ❖ whole wheat pita bread (4 Large)
- ❖ leaves lettuce (4)

Directions:

1. In a bowl, combine the artichokes, Black beans and their liquid, basil, garlic, vinegar, peppers, onion, and olives.
2. Set aside after you mix well. Slice the pita bread so that it can make a pocket. Place a lettuce in each pita and fill with the Black filling.
3. Serve.

Vegetarian Bean Curry

Servings|4   Time|55 minutes
Nutritional Content (per serving):
Cal| 531   Fat| 12g   Protein| 19g   Carbs| 19g   Fiber| 18g

Ingredients:

- vegetable oil (2 tablespoons)
- onion (1, sliced)
- curry powder (2 tablespoons, mild)
- garlic powder (1/2 teaspoon)
- ginger (1/4 teaspoon, grated)
- tomatoes (1 (15 ounces) can, seeded and diced)
- garbanzo beans (2 (15 ounces) cans)
- potatoes (2 cups, unpeeled, diced)
- carrots (1 cup, sliced)
- cauliflower pieces (1 (16 ounces) package frozen)
- peas (1 (10 ounces) package frozen)
- Water as necessary
- salt (1/4 teaspoon)
- hot brown rice (2 cups cooked)

Directions:

1. Heat up the oil over medium heat in a non-stick pan. Cook onions until softened.
2. Add curry powder, ginger and garlic powder; cook 2 minutes. Add the tomatoes, garbanzo beans, carrots, and potatoes and stir together.
3. Add cauliflower, cover and reduce heat to simmer. Cook for 20-30 minutes, until vegetable is tender, adding water if necessary.
4. Stir in peas and salt; cook 5 more minutes. Serve over hot rice.

Lunch Recipes

Fruit, Avocado & Cucumber Salad

Servings|4   Time|15 minutes
Nutritional Content (per serving):
Cal| 262   Fat| 17.1g   Protein| 3.7g   Carbs| 28.7g   Fiber| 9.5g

Ingredients:

- ❖ Large avocados (2, peeled, pitted and chopped)
- ❖ Large peach (1, peeled, pitted and chopped)
- ❖ Shallot (1, chopped finely)
- ❖ Fresh lime juice (¼ cup)
- ❖ Fresh mint (1½ tablespoons, chopped)
- ❖ Large apple (1, peeled, pitted and chopped)
- ❖ Cantaloupe (1 cup, peeled and chopped
- ❖ Seedless cucumber (1, peeled and chopped)
- ❖ Lettuce leaves (6 cups, torn)

Directions:

1. In a large salad bowl, add all the ingredients and toss to coat well.
2. Set aside for at least 10-20 minutes before serving.

Couscous, Beans & Veggie Salad

Servings|4 Time|25 minutes
Nutritional Content (per serving):
Cal| 341   Fat| 8.5g   Protein| 15.7g   Carbs| 53.2g   Fiber| 13.5g

Ingredients:
For Salad:
- ❖ Homemade vegetable broth (½ cup)
- ❖ Couscous ((½ cup)
- ❖ Canned red kidney beans (3 cups, rinsed and drained)
- ❖ Large tomatoes (2, peeled, seeded and chopped)
- ❖ Fresh spinach (5 cups, torn)

For Dressing:

- ❖ Garlic clove (1, minced)
- ❖ Shallot (¼, minced)
- ❖ Lemon zest (1½ tablespoons, grated)
- ❖ Fresh lemon juice (¼ cup)
- ❖ Extra-virgin olive oil (2 tablespoons)
- ❖ Sea salt and ground black pepper, as required

Directions:
1. In a pan, add the broth over medium heat and bring to a boil.
2. Add the couscous and stir to combine.
3. Cover the pan and immediately remove from the heat.
4. Set aside, covered for about 5-10 minutes or until all the liquid is absorbed.
5. For salad: In a large serving bowl, add the couscous and remaining ingredients and stir to combine.
6. For dressing: in another Small bowl, add all the ingredients and beat until well combined.
7. Pour the dressing over salad and gently toss to coat well.
8. Serve immediately.

Quinoa, Beans & Mango Salad

Servings|6 Time|20 minutes
Nutritional Content (per serving):
Cal| 555   Fat| 24.4g   Protein| 18.1g   Carbs| 71.5g   Fiber| 19.7g

Ingredients:

For Dressing:
- ❖ Fresh lime juice (2 tablespoons)
- ❖ Pure maple syrup (2 tablespoons)
- ❖ Dijon mustard (1 tablespoon)
- ❖ Dried thyme (½ teaspoon)
- ❖ Garlic powder (½ teaspoon)
- ❖ Onion powder (½ teaspoon)
- ❖ Ground cumin (½ teaspoon)
- ❖ Sea salt and ground black pepper, as required
- ❖ Extra-virgin olive oil (¼ cup)

For Salad:
- ❖ Fresh mango (2 cups, peeled, pitted and cubed)
- ❖ Fresh lime juice (2 tablespoons)
- ❖ Avocados (2, peeled, pitted and cubed)
- ❖ Cooked quinoa (1 cup)
- ❖ Black beans (2 (15-ounce) cans, rinsed and drained)
- ❖ Red onion (1, chopped)
- ❖ Romaine lettuce (6 cups, shredded)

Directions:

1. For dressing: in a blender, add all the ingredients except oil and pulse until well combined.
2. While the motor is running, gradually add the oil and pulse until smooth.
3. For salad: in a bowl, add the mango and 1 tablespoon of lime juice and toss to coat well.
4. In another bowl, add the avocado and remaining lime juice and toss to coat well.
5. In a large serving bowl, add the mango, avocado and remaining salad ingredients and mix.
6. Place the dressing and toss to coat well.
7. Serve immediately.

Quinoa, Beans & Veggie Salad

Servings|6   Time|15 minutes
Nutritional Content (per serving):
Cal| 354   Fat| 4.8g   Protein| 16.6g   Carbs| 62.7g   Fiber| 11.5g

Ingredients:
- Cooked quinoa (2 cups)
- Fresh baby spinach (5 cups)
- Tomato (¼ cup, peeled, seeded and chopped)
- Sea salt and ground black pepper, as required
- Canned red kidney beans (2 cups, rinsed and drained)
- Fresh dill (1½ tablespoons, chopped)
- Fresh parsley (1½ tablespoons, chopped)
- Fresh lemon juice (3 tablespoons)

Directions:
1. In a salad bowl, add all the ingredients and toss to coat well.
2. Serve immediately.

Farro & Veggies Salad

Servings|3   Time|15 minutes
Nutritional Content (per serving):
Cal| 551   Fat| 9.6g   Protein| 20.1g   Carbs| 98g   Fiber| 10.4g

Ingredients:
- Extra-virgin olive oil (2 tablespoons)
- Cooked farro (2 cups)
- Carrot (1 cup, peeled and sliced)
- Cherry tomatoes (1 cup, halved)
- Balsamic vinegar (1 tablespoon)
- Sea salt and ground black pepper, as required
- Large bell pepper (1, seeded and chopped)
- Cucumber (1 cup, chopped)
- Fresh cilantro leaves (1 teaspoon)

Directions:
1. In a Small bowl, add oil, vinegar, salt and black pepper and beat until well combined.
2. In a large bowl, add the remaining ingredients and mix well.
3. Pour the vinaigrette over salad and toss to coat well.
4. Serve immediately.

Chickpeas Stuffed Avocado

Servings|2   Time|15 minutes
Nutritional Content (per serving):
Cal| 372   Fat| 19.6g   Protein| 9.5g   Carbs| 42.9g   Fiber| 12.8g

Ingredients:

- Large avocado (1)
- Celery stalks (¼ cup, chopped)
- Small garlic clove (1, minced)
- Olive oil (½ teaspoon)
- Fresh cilantro (1 tablespoon, chopped)
- Cooked chickpeas (1¼ cups)
- Scallion (greed part) (1, sliced)
- Fresh lemon juice (1½ tablespoons)
- Sea salt and ground black pepper, as required

Directions:

1. Cut the avocado in half and then remove the pit.
2. With a spoon, scoop out the flesh from each avocado half.
3. Then, cut half of the avocado flesh in equal-sized cubes.
4. In a large bowl, add avocado cubes and remaining ingredients except for sunflower seeds and cilantro and toss to coat well.
5. Stuff each avocado half with chickpeas mixture evenly.
6. Serve immediately with the garnishing of cilantro.

Chickpeas Stuffed Sweet Potato

Servings|2 Time|55 minutes
Nutritional Content (per serving):
Cal| 286   Fat| 9.7g   Protein| 8.2g   Carbs| 43g   Fiber| 8g

Ingredients:

- Large sweet potato (1, halved lengthwise)
- Canned chickpeas (1/3 cup, rinsed and drained)
- Cooked quinoa (1/3 cup)
- Fresh cilantro (1 teaspoon, chopped)
- Olive oil (1½ tablespoons, divided)
- Sea salt and ground black pepper, as required
- Curry powder (1 teaspoon)
- Fresh lime juice (1 teaspoon)

Directions:

1. Preheat your oven to 375 degrees F.
2. Rub each sweet potato half with 1 teaspoon of oil evenly.
3. Arrange the sweet potato halves onto a baking sheet, cut side down and sprinkle with salt and black pepper.
4. Bake for approximately 40 minutes or until sweet potato becomes tender.
5. Meanwhile, for filling: in a skillet, heat the remaining oil over medium heat and cook the chickpeas, curry powder and garlic powder for about 6-8 minutes, stirring frequently.
6. Stir in the cooked quinoa, salt and black pepper and remove from the heat.
7. Remove from the oven and arrange each sweet potato halves onto a plate.
8. With a fork, fluff the flesh of each half slightly.
9. Place chickpeas mixture in each half and drizzle with lime juice
10. Serve immediately with the garnishing of cilantro and sesame seeds.

Beans & Olives Enchiladas

Servings|8 Time|35 minutes
Nutritional Content (per serving):
Cal| 358   Fat| 11.2g   Protein| 20.6g   Carbs| 46.2g   Fiber| 10.3g

Ingredients:

- Red kidney beans (1 (14-ounce) can, drained, rinsed and mashed)
- Homemade tomato paste (2 cups)
- Garlic salt (2 teaspoons)
- Whole-wheat tortillas (8)
- Cheddar cheese (2 cups, grated)
- Onion (½ cup, chopped)
- Black olives (¼ cup, pitted and sliced)

Directions:

1. Preheat your oven to 350 degrees F.
2. In a medium bowl, add the mashed beans, cheese, 1 cup of tomato paste, onions, olives and garlic salt and mix well.
3. Divide the bean mixture in 6 portions.
4. Place 1 portion of the bean mixture along center of each tortilla.
5. Roll up each tortilla and place enchiladas in large baking dish.
6. Place the remaining tomato paste on top of the filled tortillas.
7. Bake for approximately 15-20 minutes.
8. Serve warm.

Lentils with Kale

Servings|6   Time|35 minutes
Nutritional Content (per serving):
Cal| 257   Fat| 4.5g   Protein| 16.2g   Carbs| 39.3g   Fiber| 16.5g

Ingredients:

- ❖ Red lentils (1½ cups, rinsed)
- ❖ Olive oil (1½ tablespoons)
- ❖ Onion (½ cup, chopped)
- ❖ Fresh kale (6 cups, tough ends removed and chopped)
- ❖ Sea salt and ground black pepper, as required
- ❖ Homemade vegetable broth (1½ cups)
- ❖ Fresh ginger (1 teaspoon, minced)
- ❖ Garlic cloves (2, minced)
- ❖ Tomatoes (1½ cups, peeled, seeded and chopped)

Directions:

1. In a pan, add the broth and lentils over medium-high heat and bring to a boil.
2. Now adjust the heat to and simmer, covered for about 20 minutes or until almost all the liquid is absorbed.
3. Remove from the heat and set aside covered.
4. Meanwhile, in a large skillet, heat oil over medium heat and sauté the onion for about 5-6 minutes.
5. Add the ginger and garlic and sauté for about 1 minute.
6. Add tomatoes and kale and cook for about 4-5 minutes.
7. Stir in the lentils, salt and black pepper and remove from heat.
8. Serve hot.

Black Beans with Tomatoes

Servings|4   Time|40 minutes
Nutritional Content (per serving):
Cal| 327   Fat| 5.1g   Protein| 19.1g   Carbs| 54.1g   Fiber| 18.8g

Ingredients:

- ❖ Olive oil (1 tablespoon)
- ❖ Garlic cloves (5, chopped finely)
- ❖ Ground cumin (1 teaspoon)
- ❖ Tomatoes (2 cups, peeled, seeded and chopped)
- ❖ Homemade vegetable broth (½ cup)
- ❖ Small onions (2, chopped)
- ❖ Dried oregano (1 teaspoon)
- ❖ Sea salt and ground black pepper, as required
- ❖ Black beans (2 (13½-ounce) cans, rinsed and drained)

Directions:

1. Heat the olive oil in a pan over medium heat and cook the onion for about 5-7 minutes, stirring frequently.
2. Add garlic, oregano, spices, salt and black pepper and cook for about 1 minute.
3. Add the tomatoes and cook for about 1-2 minutes.
4. Add in the beans and broth and bring to a boil.
5. Now, adjust the heat to medium-low and simmer, covered for about 15 minutes.
6. Serve hot.

Chickpeas with Swiss Chard

Servings|4 Time|30 minutes
Nutritional Content (per serving):
Cal| 260   Fat| 8.6g   Protein| 12g   Carbs| 34g   Fiber| 9g

Ingredients:

- ❖ Olive oil (2 tablespoons)
- ❖ Garlic cloves (4, minced)
- ❖ Dried oregano (1 teaspoon, crushed)
- ❖ Tomato (1 cup, peeled, seeded and chopped finely)
- ❖ Swiss chard (5 cups, chopped)
- ❖ Fresh lemon juice (2 tablespoons)
- ❖ Fresh basil (1 teaspoon, chopped)

- ❖ Medium onion (1, chopped)
- ❖ Dried thyme (1 teaspoon, crushed)
- ❖ Paprika (½ teaspoon)
- ❖ Canned chickpeas (2½ cups, rinsed and drained)
- ❖ Filtered water (2 tablespoons)
- ❖ Sea salt and ground black pepper, as required

Directions:

1. In a skillet, heat the olive oil over medium heat and sauté the onion for about 6-8 minutes.
2. Add the garlic, herbs and paprika and sauté for about 1 minute.
3. Add the Swiss chard and (2 tablespoons) of water and cook for about 2-3 minutes.
4. Add the tomatoes and chickpeas and cook for about 2-3 minutes.
5. Add in the lemon juice, salt and black pepper and remove from the heat.
6. Serve hot with the garnishing of basil.

Chickpea Balls in Tomato Sauce

Servings|6   Time|35 minutes
Nutritional Content (per serving):
Cal| 243   Fat| 7g   Protein| 10.4g   Carbs| 39.1g   Fiber| 9.9g

Ingredients:

- ❖ Cooked chickpeas (1½ cups)
- ❖ Onions (½ cup, chopped)
- ❖ Green bell pepper (¼ cup, seeded and chopped)
- ❖ Cayenne powder (½ teaspoon)
- ❖ Chickpea flour (½-1 cup)
- ❖ Olive oil (2 tablespoons)
- ❖ Fresh button mushrooms (2 cups)
- ❖ Fresh oregano (1 teaspoon)
- ❖ Fresh basil (1 teaspoon)
- ❖ Sea salt, as required
- ❖ Homemade tomato sauce (6 cups)

Directions:

1. In a food processor, add the chickpeas, veggies, herbs and spices and pulse until well combined.
2. Transfer the mixture into a large bowl with flour and mix until well combined.
3. Make desired-sized balls from the mixture.
4. In a skillet, heat the grapeseed oil over medium-high heat and cook the balls in 2 batches for about 4-5 minutes or until golden brown from all sides.
5. In a large pan, add the tomato sauce and veggie balls over medium heat and simmer for about 5 minutes.
6. Serve hot.

Chipotle Black Bean Chili

Servings|4   Time|40 minutes
Nutritional Content (per serving):
Cal| 60   Fat| 4g   Protein| 1g   Carbs| 6g   Fiber| 2g

Ingredients:

- olive oil (1 tablespoon)
- onion (1 cup, finely chopped)
- cloves garlic (4, minced)
- chipotle powder (1/2 teaspoon)
- cumin (1/2 teaspoon)
- salt (1/4 teaspoon)
- black beans (1 (30 ounces) can, drained and rinsed)
- tomatoes (1 (28 ounces) can, diced and seedless)
- Fresh cilantro (1 teaspoon)

Directions:

1. In a large non-stick pan, heat olive oil over medium heat. Add onions and garlic and cook 5 minutes or until they are soft.
2. Add in your tomatoes, beans, salt, cumin and chipotle powder then allow to boil.
3. Switch your heat to low, cover and allow to simmer until chili thickens (about 20 mins). Garnish with fresh cilantro. Serve.

Quinoa Stew

Servings|4   Time|55 minutes
Nutritional Content (per serving):
Cal| 240   Fat| 4g   Protein| 14g   Carbs| 38g   Fiber| 17g

Ingredients:

- ❖ vegetable oil (1 tablespoon)
- ❖ onion (1 Large, chopped)
- ❖ cloves garlic (2, finely chopped)
- ❖ green bell pepper (1 med, chopped)
- ❖ water (3 cups or broth)

- ❖ Quinoa (1 1/4 cups, uncooked, rinsed)
- ❖ tomato sauce (1 can)
- ❖ oregano (½ teaspoon)
- ❖ thyme (½ teaspoon)
- ❖ basil (½ teaspoon)
- ❖ paprika (½ teaspoon)

Directions:

1. Heat the oil up over medium heat in a saucepan. Cook onion, bell pepper, and garlic, stir often, until vegetables are tender.
2. Stir in water, Quinoa, tomato sauce and spices.
3. Turn the heat down low and cover it partially and let simmer 40 minutes or until Quinoa are tender.
4. Serve.

Vegetable Couscous

Servings|4 Time|10 minutes
Nutritional Content (per serving):
Cal| 396   Fat| 18g   Protein| 12g   Carbs| 48g   Fiber| 6g

Ingredients:

- vegetable stock (1 1/2 cups)
- couscous (1 cup, plain)
- olive oil (4 tablespoons, divided)
- red onion (1, chopped)
- cloves garlic (2, minced)
- tomatoes (3 Large, seeded and diced)
- yellow bell pepper (1, seeded and chopped)
- red bell pepper (1, seeded and chopped)
- Zucchinis (2, seeded and chopped)
- peas (1 cup, frozen and thawed)
- balsamic vinegar (2 tablespoons)
- feta cheese (2 tablespoons, crumbled)

Directions:

1. In a saucepan, over high heat, bring a tablespoons of olive oil and vegetable stock to a boil. Remove from heat and stir in couscous.
2. Cover and let sit for 5-10 minutes.
3. In another pan over medium heat, add the remaining oil and cook the garlic and onions until softened.
4. Mix in the Zucchini, tomatoes and bell peppers then continue to stir until tender.
5. Stir in your peas and continue to cook for another 3 more minutes.
6. Add in your cheese and vinegar then toss to combine.
7. Pour the vegetable mixture over couscous. Serve.

Quinoa Spaghetti Stew

Servings|4   Time|1 hour
Nutritional Content (per serving):
Cal| 393   Fat| 12g   Protein| 18g   Carbs| 55g   Fiber| 17g

Ingredients:

- olive oil (3 tablespoons)
- onion (1 Large, chopped)
- cloves garlic (4, minced)
- carrots (3, chopped)
- celery stalks (3, chopped)
- Quinoa (1 cup, uncooked)
- water (2 1/2 quarts)
- salt (2 teaspoons)
- bay leaf (1)
- linguine (1/4 pound, broken into 1 1/2-inch pieces)
- kale (2 cups, chopped)
- Italian parsley (1/2 cup, chopped)

Directions:

1. Heat the olive oil over moderate heat in a pot. Cook the onion, garlic, and carrots and celery for 10 minutes, stirring occasionally, until tender.
2. Add the Quinoa, water, salt, and bay leaf to the pot. Bring to a boil.
3. Turn the heat down so that the content can simmer, cover the pot partially, stir often for 15 minutes.
4. Add the linguine and let it simmer, stir often, cook the Quinoa, kale and pasta until they are tender, 15 to 20 minutes longer.
5. Stir parsley into the stew. Serve

Quinoa Stir Fry

Servings|4 Time|23 minutes
Nutritional Content (per serving):
Cal| 91 Fat| 5g   Protein| 3g   Carbs| 10g   Fiber| 4g

Ingredients:

- sugar snap peas (1 cup)
- olive oil (2 tablespoons)
- onion (1 Small, chopped)
- mushrooms (8 ounces, sliced)
- artichoke hearts (1 (8 ounces) can, drained)
- green Quinoa (1 (8 ounces) can, drained)
- half and half cream (4 tablespoons)
- salt (1/2 teaspoon)

Directions:

1. Bring a Small saucepan of water to boil. Once the water is boiling add sugar snap peas and add the salt. Once you do that make sure to turn off the heat and wait for 5 minutes. Drain the sugar snap peas under the water and set aside.
2. Drain the content under cold water, dry it with paper towel. Set aside.
3. In a pan heat an oil of your choice (I like to use olive oil) and fry onions for 4-5 minutes. Add mushrooms as well and stir for another 3-4 minutes.
4. Add sugar snap peas, artichoke and lentils while also adding cream, salt and pepper and fry for another 2-3 minutes.
5. Voila, ready to serve.

Grilled Vegetable Quesadillas

Servings|2-4 Time|20 minutes
Nutritional Content (per serving):
Cal| 57 Fat| 1g Protein| 4g Carbs| 12g Fiber| 3g

Ingredients:

- Zucchini (1 Small)
- yellow squash (1 Small)
- yellow onion (1 Small)
- red pepper (1, seeded)
- Portobello mushroom (1 Small)

- oregano (1/2 teaspoon)
- salt (1/4 teaspoon)
- whole wheat tortillas (2)
- low fat Mozzarella cheese (1/2 cup, shredded)

Directions:
1. Over medium heat grill vegetables until all of the vegetables are cooked.
2. Season with oregano and salt.
3. Slice vegetables and toss together. Heat a non-stick pan sprayed with non-stick cooking spray over medium heat and place one tortilla in the pan.
4. Spread some of the vegetable mixture over the tortilla, sprinkle with cheese and top with the remaining tortilla.
5. Turn tortilla over and heat the other side until cheese melts but do not brown the tortillas. Serve.

Quick Broccoli Pasta

Servings|2 Time|16 minutes
Nutritional Content (per serving):
Cal| 246   Fat| 11g   Protein| 11g   Carbs| 29g   Fiber| 5g

Ingredients:

- ❖ broccoli florets (2 cups)
- ❖ whole wheat pasta (1/2 pound)
- ❖ extra virgin olive oil (1/2 tablespoons)
- ❖ parmesan cheese (1 1/2 tablespoons, grated)
- ❖ garlic powder (1/8 teaspoon)

Directions:

1. Bring a salted water to boil in a pot. Add in pasta and broccoli then cook until tender (about 8 minutes).
2. Drain well. In a large shallow pasta bowl put the pasta mixture and toss with olive oil, garlic powder and cheese. Serve.

Caribbean Rice & Pea

Servings|4-6 Time|30 minutes
Nutritional Content (per serving):
Cal| 164 Fat| 3g Protein| 9g Carbs| 27g Fiber| 7g

Ingredients:

- olive oil (1 tablespoon)
- onion (1 Medium, chopped)
- sticks celery (2, chopped)
- cloves garlic (2, chopped)
- tomato paste (1 (14 ounces) can)
- oregano (1/2 teaspoon)
- thyme (1/2 teaspoon)
- vegetable stock (1(14 ounces) can)
- red beans (1 (28 ounces) can, drained and rinsed)

Directions:

1. In a large non-stick pan, heat olive oil over medium heat. Cook onions, celery and garlic stirring until just tender.
2. Stir in tomato paste, oregano and thyme. Add stock, stir and bring to a boil.
3. Simmer uncovered about 15 minutes or until mixture thickens. Add red beans and let cook until heated through. Serve over rice.

Quinoa Risotto

Servings|4   Time|25 minutes
Nutritional Content (per serving)
Cal| 457   Fat| 9g   Protein| 21g   Carbs| 73g   Fiber| 17g

Ingredients:

- Olive oil (2 tablespoons)
- cloves garlic (3, minced)
- vegetable stock (3 cups) brown rice (1 1/4 cup)
- Quinoa (1 cup, cooked)
- Fresh parmesan cheese (1/4 cup, grated)

- leeks (4 Medium, chopped)
- red bell pepper (1 medium, seeded, finely chopped)
- basil (1 tablespoon, chopped)
- Italian parsley (1/4 cup, chopped)

Directions:

1. In a large pot, heat olive oil over moderate heat and cook leeks, garlic, and red bell pepper until softened.
2. Add stock along with the rice, and basil. Cover and let simmer until rice is done then add cooked Quinoa and stir for 10 minutes.
3. Remove from heat and add parsley and parmesan cheese. Serve.

Mushroom and Beans Stew

Servings|4   Time|27 minutes
Nutritional Content (per serving)
Cal| 261   Fat| 9g   Protein| 15g   Carbs| 33g   Fiber| 13g

Ingredients:
- olive oil (2 tablespoons)
- onions (1 cup, chopped)
- dried thyme (3/4 teaspoon)
- stewed tomatoes (1 (14 ounces) can, chopped)
- white mushrooms (1 pound, sliced)
- garlic (1 teaspoon, minced)
- vegetable stock (2 (14 ounces) cans)
- dry white wine (1/4 cup)
- cannellini beans (30 ounces, canned)

Directions:
1. Heat up the oil over medium heat in a saucepan. Cook the mushrooms, onion, thyme and garlic for about 7 minutes.
2. Bring to a boil when you add vegetable stock, wine and tomatoes.
3. Cover and simmer for about 15 additional minutes. In a bowl, mash up at least 1 cup of the beans until it has a smooth consistency; add the mashed beans into the stew.
4. Stir the rest of the beans, heat until hot. Serve immediately.

Quinoa & Brown Rice Bowl

Servings|6   Time|47 minutes
Nutritional Content (per serving):
Cal| 307   Fat| 7g   Protein| 14g   Carbs| 48g   Fiber| 12g

Ingredients:
- olive oil (2 tablespoons)
- carrots (2, finely chopped)
- garlic clove (1, minced)
- dried sage (1 teaspoon)
- vegetable stock (3 cups)
- onion (1, chopped)
- bell pepper (1, chopped)
- dried basil (1 tablespoon)
- brown rice (1 cup)
- Quinoa (1 cup, uncooked and rinsed)

Directions:
1. Heat up the olive oil over medium heat in a pan. Cook pepper onion and carrot until soft (about 6 minutes).
2. Add garlic and cook for one more minute. Add basil, sage and rice. Stir to combine.
3. Stir in broth. Bring to a boil, stirring occasionally. Add Quinoa.
4. Close the lid then switch to low heat. Simmer for another 20 minutes. Fluff with fork and serve.

Vegetarian Rice Casserole

Servings|4 Time|50 minutes
Nutritional Content (per serving)
Cal| 57   Fat| 1g   Protein| 4g   Carbs| 9g   Fiber| 2g

Ingredients:

- Non-stick cooking spray
- Fresh mushrooms (1/4 cup, sliced)
- carrots (1/4 cup, chopped)
- onion (1/4 cup, finely chopped)
- salt (1 teaspoon)
- oregano (1 teaspoon)
- fat-free cheddar cheese (1/4 cup, shredded)
- long-grain brown rice (1 cup)
- broccoli (1/4 cup, chopped)
- red bell pepper (1/4 cup, seeded and chopped)
- paprika (1 teaspoon)
- vegetable stock (2 -1/2 cups)

Directions:

1. Preheat oven to 425 degrees. Lightly grease a glass baking dish (13x9) with cooking spray.
2. Mix the broccoli, brown rice, carrots, mushrooms, bell pepper, salt, onion, paprika, oregano, and broth.
3. Mix well and cover with foil. Bake until cooked through (about 30 minutes); stirring when the baking is halfway.
4. Add the cheese on top and allow it to melt prior to serving.

Dinner Recipes

Turkey & Lentil Soup

Servings|8 Time|1 hour 25 minutes
Nutritional Content (per serving):
Cal| 485   Fat| 16.5g   Protein| 43g   Carbs| 44.6g   Fiber| 16.6g

Ingredients:

- Olive oil (2 tablespoons)
- Sea salt and ground black pepper, as required
- Large celery stalk (1, chopped)
- Garlic cloves (6, chopped)
- Large potatoes (2, peeled and chopped
- Tomatoes (4 cups, peeled, seeded and chopped)
- Ground turkey (1½ pounds)
- Large carrot (1, peeled and chopped)
- Large onion (1, chopped)
- Dried rosemary (1 teaspoon)
- Chicken bone broth (8-9 cups)
- Dry lentils (2 cups)
- Fresh parsley (1½ tablespoons, chopped)

Directions:

1. In a large soup pan, heat the olive oil over medium-high heat and cook the turkey for about 5 minutes or until browned.
2. With a slotted spoon, transfer the turkey into a bowl and set aside.
3. In the same pan, add the carrot, celery onion, garlic and dried herbs over medium heat and cook for about 5 minutes.
4. Add the potatoes and cook for about 4-5 minutes.
5. Add the cooked turkey, tomatoes and broth and bring to a boil over high heat.
6. Now adjust the heat to low and cook, covered for about 10 minutes.
7. Add the lentils and cook, covered for about 40 minutes.
8. Stir in black pepper and remove from the heat.
9. Serve hot with the garnishing of parsley.

Lentil & Sweet Potato Soup

Servings|4   Time|1 hour 5 minutes
Nutritional Content (per serving):
Cal| 471   Fat| 5.6g   Protein| 19.3g   Carbs| 61g   Fiber| 19.7g

Ingredients:

- Olive oil (1 tablespoon)
- Carrots (½ cup, peeled and chopped)
- Homemade vegetable broth (4½ cups)
- Red lentils (1 cup, rinsed)
- Sea salt and ground black pepper, as required
- Onion (1 cup, chopped)
- Celery (½ cup, chopped)
- Garlic cloves (2, minced)
- Sweet potatoes (2½ cups, peeled and chopped)
- Fresh lemon juice (1½ tablespoons)
- Fresh cilantro (1 teaspoon, chopped)

Directions:

1. In a large Dutch oven, heat the oil over medium heat and sauté the onion, carrot and celery for about 5-7 minutes.
2. Add the garlic and sauté for about 1 minute.
3. Add the sweet potatoes and cook for about 1-2 minutes.
4. Add in the broth and bring to a boil.
5. Now adjust the heat to low and simmer, covered for about 5 minutes.
6. Stir in the red lentils and gain bring to a boil over medium-high heat.
7. Now adjust the heat to low and simmer, covered for about 25-30 minutes or until desired doneness.
8. Stir in the lemon juice, salt and black pepper and remove from the heat.
9. Serve hot with the garnishing of cilantro.

Beans & Sweet Potato Soup

Servings|6   Time|1 hour
Nutritional Content (per serving):
Cal| 411   Fat| 5.7g   Protein| 22.7g   Carbs| 65.7g   Fiber| 18.9g

Ingredients:

- Olive oil (2 tablespoons)
- Large sweet potato (½, peeled and cubed)
- Celery stalks (2, chopped)
- Large tomatoes (2, peeled, seeded and chopped finely)
- Red kidney beans (1 (15-ounce) can, rinsed and drained)
- Black beans (½ (15-ounce) can, drained and rinsed)
- Fresh cilantro (¼ cup, chopped)
- Large onion (½, chopped)
- Large carrot (1, peeled and chopped)
- Garlic cloves (2, minced)
- Great Northern beans (1 (15-ounce) can, rinsed and drained)
- Homemade vegetable broth(6 cups)
- Sea salt and ground black pepper, as required

Directions:

1. In a Dutch oven, heat the oil over medium heat and sauté the onion, sweet potato, carrot and celery for about 6-8 minutes.
2. Add the garlic and sauté for about 1 minute.
3. Add in the tomatoes and cook for about 2-3 minutes.
4. Add the beans and broth and bring to a boil over medium-high heat.
5. Cover the pan with lid and cook for about 25-30 minutes.
6. Stir in the cilantro and remove from heat.
7. Serve hot.

Pasta & Beans Stew

Servings|6 Time|50 minutes
Nutritional Content (per serving):
Cal| 314   Fat| 10g   Protein| 14.4g   Carbs| 46g   Fiber| 2.31g

Ingredients:

- Olive oil (¼ cup)
- Fresh mushrooms (8 ounces, sliced)
- Garlic (2 tablespoons, chopped finely)
- Homemade vegetable broth (4½ cups)
- Apple cider vinegar (2 tablespoons)
- Cannellini beans (1 (15-ounce) can, drained and rinsed)
- Large onion (1, chopped)
- Large tomatoes (2, peeled, seeded and chopped)
- Dried mixed herbs (1½ tablespoons)
- Whole-wheat fusilli pasta (1 cup)
- Nutritional yeast (1/3 cup)
- Sea salt and ground black pepper, as required

Directions:

1. In a large pan, heat the oil over medium heat and sauté the onion, mushrooms, potato and tomato for about 4-5 minutes.
2. Add the garlic, bay leaves and herbs and sauté for about 1 minute.
3. Add the broth and bring to a boil.
4. Stir in the vinegar, pasta and nutritional yeast and again bring to a boil.
5. Now adjust the heat to medium-low and simmer, covered for about 20 minutes.
6. Stir in the greens and beans and simmer, uncovered for about 4-5 minutes.
7. Stir in the salt and black pepper and serve hot.

Barley & Lentil Stew

Servings|8   Time|1 hour 10 minutes
Nutritional Content (per serving):
Cal| 264   Fat| 5.8g   Protein| 14.3g   Carbs| 41.1g   Fiber| 14.1g

Ingredients:

- Olive oil (2 tablespoons)
- Large onion (1, chopped)
- Garlic cloves (2, minced)
- Ground cumin (1½ tablespoons)
- red lentils (1 cup)
- Homemade vegetable broth (5-6 cups)
- Fresh spinach (6 cups, torn)
- Carrots (2, peeled and chopped)
- Celery stalks (2, chopped)
- Ground coriander (1½ tablespoons)
- Barley (1 cup)
- Tomatoes (5 cups, peeled, seeded and chopped finely)
- Sea salt and ground black pepper, as required

Directions:

1. In a large pan, heat the oil over medium heat and sauté the carrots, onion, celery and celery for about 5 minutes.
2. Add the garlic and spices and sauté for about 1 minute.
3. Add the barley, lentils, tomatoes and broth and bring to a rolling boil.
4. Now adjust the heat to low and simmer, covered for about 40 minutes.
5. Stir in the spinach, salt and black pepper and simmer for about 3-4 minutes.
6. Serve hot.

Turkey & Beans Chili

Servings|6   Time|1 hour
Nutritional Content (per serving):
Cal| 366   Fat| 11.2g   Protein| 28.7g   Carbs| 40.6g   Fiber| 13.4g

Ingredients:

- Olive oil (2 tablespoons)
- Onion (1, chopped)
- Lean ground turkey (1 pound)
- Tomatoes (3 cups, peeled, seeded and chopped finely
- Black beans (1 (15-ounce) can, rinsed and drained), rinsed and drained
- Bell pepper (1, seeded and chopped)
- Garlic cloves (2, chopped)
- Filtered water (2 cups)
- Ground cumin (1 teaspoon)
- Red kidney beans (1 (15-ounce) can, rinsed and drained)

Directions:

1. In a large Dutch oven, heat the olive oil over medium-low heat and sauté bell pepper, onion and garlic for about 5 minutes.
2. Add the turkey and cook for about 5-6 minutes, breaking up the chunks with a wooden spoon.
3. Add the water, tomatoes and spices and bring to a boil over high heat.
4. Now adjust the heat to medium-low and stir in beans and corn.
5. Simmer, covered for about 30 minutes, stirring occasionally.
6. Serve hot.

Three Beans Chili

Servings|6   Time|1¼ hours
Nutritional Content (per serving):
Cal| 342   Fat| 6.1g   Protein| 20.3g   Carbs| 56g   Fiber| 21.3g

Ingredients:

- ❖ Olive oil (2 tablespoons)
- ❖ Celery stalks (2, chopped)
- ❖ Garlic cloves (3, minced)
- ❖ Red chili powder (1½ tablespoons)
- ❖ Tomatoes (2 pounds, peeled, seeded and chopped finely)
- ❖ Water (4½ cups)
- ❖ Red kidney beans (1 (15-ounce) can, rinsed and drained)
- ❖ Bell pepper (1, seeded and chopped)
- ❖ Scallion (1, chopped)
- ❖ Dried oregano (1 teaspoon, crushed)
- ❖ Sea salt and ground black pepper, as required
- ❖ Cannellini beans (1 (15-ounce) can , rinsed and drained)
- ❖ Black beans (½ (15-ounce) can, rinsed and drained)

Directions:

1. In a large pan, heat the oil over medium heat and cook the bell peppers, celery, scallion and garlic for about 8-10 minutes, stirring frequently.
2. Add the oregano, spices, salt, black pepper, tomatoes and water and bring to a boil.
3. Simmer for about 20 minutes.
4. Stir in the beans and simmer for about 30 minutes.
5. Serve hot.

Pasta & Chickpeas Curry

Servings|6 Time|55 minutes
Nutritional Content (per serving):
Cal| 338   Fat| 5.9g   Protein| 15.1g   Carbs| 58.4g   Fiber| 10.3g

Ingredients:

- Whole-wheat pasta (10 ounces)
- Medium onion (1, chopped)
- Dried basil (1 teaspoon, crushed)
- Tomatoes (2 pounds, peeled, seeded and chopped)
- Medium red bell pepper (1, seeded and sliced thinly)
- Chickpeas (1 (15-ounce) can, drained and rinsed)
- Olive oil (1 tablespoon)
- Garlic cloves (3, minced)
- Curry powder (1½ tablespoons)
- Cauliflower (4 cups, cut into bite-sized pieces)
- Filtered water (1 cup)
- Fresh baby spinach (1 cup)
- Fresh parsley (1½ tablespoons, chopped)
- Sea salt, as required

Directions:

1. In a pan of the salted boiling water, add the pasta and cook for about 8-10 minutes or according to package's directions.
2. Drain the pasta well and set aside.
3. Heat the oil in a large cast-iron skillet over medium heat and sauté the onion for about 4-5 minutes.
4. Add the garlic, basil and curry powder and sauté for about 1 minute.
5. Stir in the tomatoes, cauliflower, bell pepper and water and bring to a gentle boil.
6. Now adjust the heat to medium-low and simmer, covered for about 20 minutes.
7. Stir in the chickpeas and cook for about 5 minutes.
8. Add the spinach and cook for about 3-4 minutes.
9. Stir in the pasta and remove from the heat.
10. Serve hot.

Lentils, Apple & Veggie Curry

Servings|8   Time|1¾ hours
Nutritional Content (per serving):
Cal| 263   Fat| 2.9g   Protein| 14.7g   Carbs| 47g   Fiber| 20g

Ingredients:

- ❖ Water (8 cups)
- ❖ Red lentils (2 cups, rinsed)
- ❖ Large white onion (1, chopped)
- ❖ Large tomatoes (2, peeled, seeded and chopped)
- ❖ Pumpkin (3 cups, peeled, seeded and cubed into cubes)
- ❖ Sea salt and ground black pepper, as required
- ❖ Ground turmeric (½ teaspoon)
- ❖ Olive oil (1 tablespoon)
- ❖ Garlic cloves (3, minced)
- ❖ Curry powder (1½ tablespoons)
- ❖ Carrots (3, peeled and chopped)
- ❖ Granny smith apple (1, cored and chopped)
- ❖ Fresh spinach (2 cups, chopped)

Directions:

1. In a pan, add the water, turmeric and lentils over high heat and bring to a boil.
2. Now adjust the heat to medium-low and simmer, covered for about 30 minutes.
3. Drain the lentils, reserving 2½ cups of the cooking liquid.
4. Meanwhile, in another large pan, heat the oil over medium heat and sauté the onion for about 2-3 minutes.
5. Add in the garlic and sauté for about 1 minute.
6. Add the tomatoes and cook for about 5 minutes.
7. Stir in the curry powder and spices and cook for about 1 minute.
8. Add the carrots, potatoes, pumpkin, cooked lentils and reserved cooking liquid and bring to a gentle boil.
9. Now adjust the heat to medium-low and simmer, covered for about 40-45 minutes or until desired doneness of the vegetables.
10. Stir in the apple and spinach and simmer for about 15 minutes.
11. Stir in the salt and black pepper and remove from the heat.
12. Serve hot.

Beans & Veggies Pilaf

Servings|4   Time|1¼ hours
Nutritional Content (per serving)
Cal| 463   Fat| 10.1g   Protein| 18.5g   Carbs| 76.7g   Fiber| 11.6g

Ingredients:

- ❖ Olive oil (2 tablespoons)
- ❖ Fresh mushrooms (2 cups, sliced)
- ❖ Sea salt and ground black pepper, as required
- ❖ Scallions (4, chopped)
- ❖ Fresh parsley (1 teaspoon, chopped)
- ❖ Garlic cloves (2, minced)
- ❖ Brown rice (1¼ cups, rinsed)
- ❖ Homemade vegetable broth (2 cups)
- ❖ Bell pepper (1, seeded and chopped)
- ❖ Canned red kidney beans (16 ounces, drained and rinsed)

Directions:

1. In a large saucepan, heat the oil over medium heat and sauté the onion for about 4-5 minutes.
2. Add the garlic and mushrooms and cook about 5-6 minutes.
3. Stir in the rice and cook for about 1-2 minutes, stirring continuously.
4. Stir in the broth, salt and black pepper and bring to a boil.
5. Now adjust the heat to low and simmer, covered for about 35 minutes, stirring occasionally.
6. Add in the bell pepper and beans and cook for about 5-10 minutes or until all the liquid is absorbed.
7. Serve hot with the garnishing of parsley.

Rice, Lentil & Veggie Casserole

Servings|6   Time|1¼ hours
Nutritional Content (per serving):
Cal| 192   Fat| 1.8g   Protein| 11.3g   Carbs| 34.5g   Fiber| 12g

Ingredients:

- Water (2½ cups, divided)
- Wild rice (½ cup, rinsed)
- Small onion (1, chopped)
- Zucchini (1/3 cup, peeled, seeded and chopped)
- Celery stalk (1/3 cup, chopped)
- Large tomato (1, peeled, seeded and chopped)
- Dried oregano (1 teaspoon, crushed)

- Red lentils (1 cup, rinsed)
- Olive oil (1 teaspoon)
- Garlic cloves (3, minced)
- Carrot (1/3 cup, peeled and chopped)
- Tomato paste (8 ounces)
- Sea salt and ground black pepper, as required

Directions:

1. In a saucepan, add 1 cup of the water and rice over medium-high heat and bring to a rolling boil.
2. Now adjust the heat to low and simmer, covered for about 20 minutes.
3. Meanwhile, in another pan, add the remaining water and lentils over medium heat and bring to a rolling boil.
4. Now adjust the heat to low and simmer, covered for about 15 minutes.
5. Transfer the cooked rice and lentils into a casserole dish and set aside.
6. Preheat your oven to 350 degrees F.
7. Heat the oil in a large skillet over medium heat and sauté the onion and garlic for about 4-5 minutes.
8. Add the Zucchini, carrot, celery, tomato and tomato paste and cook for about 4-5 minutes.
9. Stir in the oregano, salt and black pepper and remove from the heat.
10. Transfer the vegetable mixture into the casserole dish with rice and lentils and stir to combine.
11. Bake for approximately 30 minutes.
12. Serve hot.

Pasta with Quinoa Sauce

Servings|4   Time|2¼ hours
Nutritional Content (per serving):
Cal| 510   Fat| 23g   Protein| 17.1g   Carbs| 71g   Fiber| 6.5g

Ingredients:

- Olive oil (5 tablespoons, divided)
- Carrot (1, peeled and chopped finely)
- Mushrooms (3 cups, chopped)
- Dried mixed herbs (1½ tablespoons)
- Tomatoes (2 cups, peeled, seeded and crushed)
- Balsamic vinegar (1 tablespoon)
- Sea salt and ground black pepper, as required
- Celery stalks (3, chopped finely)
- Onion (1, chopped finely)
- Quinoa (1 cup, rinsed)
- 4 garlic cloves, chopped
- Homemade vegetable broth (1½ cups)
- Water (½-1 cup)
- Nutritional yeast (2 tablespoons)
- Oat milk (¼ cup)
- Whole-wheat pasta (¾ pound)

Directions:

1. Preheat your oven to 300 degrees F.
2. In a large Dutch oven, heat 3 tablespoons of the olive oil over medium heat and cook the celery, carrots and onion for about 10 minutes, stirring frequently.
3. Stir in the quinoa and cook for about 3 minutes.
4. Add the remaining oil and mushrooms and stir to combine.
5. Now adjust the heat to medium-high and cook for about 5 minutes.
6. Add the garlic and dried herbs and cook for about 1-2 minutes.
7. Add the broth and cook for about 5 minutes.
8. Add the tomatoes, water and vinegar and bring to a boil.
9. Remove the Dutch oven from heat and transfer into the oven.
10. Bake, uncovered for about 1½ hours, stirring once after 1 hour.
11. Meanwhile, in a pan of the lightly salted boiling water, cook the pasta for about 8-10 minutes or according to package's instructions.
12. Remove the Dutch oven from oven and stir in the nutritional yeast and oat milk.
13. Drin the pasta well and divide onto serving plates.
14. Top with Bolognese sauce and serve.

Chicken Lettuce Wraps

Servings|2   Time|15 minutes
Nutritional Content (per serving)
Cal| 338   Fat| 10g   Protein| 26g   Carbs| 39g   Fiber| 9g

Ingredients:

- ❖ Mayonnaise (1/4 cup, low fat)
- ❖ white beans (1/2 cup, canned, cooked, drained)
- ❖ chicken breast strips (1/2 pound cooked, preferably grilled)
- ❖ lemon juice (2 teaspoons)
- ❖ feta cheese (1/3 cup, crumbled)
- ❖ pimentos (2 tablespoons, chopped)
- ❖ lettuce leaves (8 Large, washed, and dried)

Directions:

1. In a medium bowl, combine mayonnaise and lemon juice.
2. Stir in beans, mashing slightly with fork.
3. Add cheese and pimentos and mix lightly.
4. Spread lettuce leaves evenly with bean mixture.
5. Top with chicken; roll up.
6. Serve.

Couscous with Turkey

Servings|4 Time|46 minutes
Nutritional Content (per serving)
Cal| 469 Fat| 24g Protein| 18g Carbs| 40g Fiber| 4g

Ingredients:

- extra-virgin olive oil (4 tablespoons)
- onion (1, chopped)
- cloves garlic (3, minced)
- smoked paprika (1 teaspoon)
- salt (1/2 teaspoon)
- turkey stock (4 cups, divided)
- butter (2 tablespoons)
- Italian parsley (1/2 cup, chopped)
- turkey thighs (1 pound boneless, skinless, chopped)
- carrots (1 cup, shredded)
- Ground cinnamon (1/8 teaspoon)
- dried fruits (1 cup chopped, pitted dates, apricots)
- couscous (1 1/2 cups)

Directions:

1. Set your oil to get hot on medium heat. Cook turkey and brown 3 to 4 minutes on each side.
2. Add onions, garlic, carrots, and season with spices and salt. Cook 6-8 minutes.
3. Stir the fruits into the turkey and vegetables, and 2 ½ cups of stock.
4. Allow to boil. Turn down the heat to low, cover and let it simmer for 10 minutes.
5. In a separate Small saucepan, over medium heat, pour 1 ½ cups of stock and bring up to a boil then stir in the couscous.
6. Take the content off the heat and let it stand 5 minutes while the cover is on. Fluff with fork and serve with turkey.

Easy Turkey Chili

Servings|4-6 Time|1 hour 12 minutes
Nutritional Content (per serving)
Cal| 193   Fat| 13g   Protein| 16g   Carbs| 5g   Fiber| 1g

Ingredients:

- olive oil (3 tablespoons)
- onion (1 medium, chopped)
- Ground cumin (1 teaspoon)
- tomato (1, seeded and chopped)
- Pork broth (1 cup)
- salt (1 teaspoon)
- garlic cloves (4, minced)
- bay leaf (1)
- dried oregano (1 teaspoon)
- tomato sauce (1 (14 ounces) can)
- red beans (2 (14 ounces) cans, drained and rinsed)

Directions:

1. Heat the oil over medium heat, in a large pot and cook the onions and garlic for 5 minutes.
2. Turn the heat from Medium to high. Add oregano, bay leaf, turkey and cumin. Cook for 5-7 minutes or until turkey has browned.
3. Add broth, tomato sauce, tomato and salt. Once the pot is boiling, lower the heat to simmer. Let it simmer for about 20 minutes, covered.
4. If needed, add more water and beans and continue to simmer for 15 more minutes. Serve.

Ham, Bean and Cabbage Stew

Servings|3   Time|32 minutes
Nutritional Content (per serving)
Cal| 543   Fat| 21g   Protein| 40g   Carbs| 47g   Fiber| 8g

Ingredients:

- extra virgin olive oil (1 tablespoon)
- onion (1 Large, chopped)
- cloves garlic (5, chopped finely)
- tomatoes (1 (28 ounces) can, seedless, drained)
- kidney beans (2 (14 ounces) cans)
- dried rosemary (1 teaspoon)
- smoked ham (8 ounces, chopped)
- stalks celery (2, sliced)
- chicken broth (4 cups)
- whole wheat pasta (3 cups)
- coleslaw (8 ounces)
- dried basil (1 teaspoon)

Directions:

1. In a good size pot, heat olive oil over medium heat. Cook ham, onion, celery and garlic stirring occasionally, until vegetables are tender.
2. Stir in broth and tomatoes, breaking up tomatoes. Stir the pasta in, heat to boiling and turn down the heat low.
3. Cover and simmer about 10 minutes or until pasta is tender. Stir in coleslaw, beans, basil and oregano.
4. Bring stew to a boil and reduce heat to low. Simmer uncovered about 5-7 minutes or until cabbage is tender.

Grilled Fish Tacos

Servings|4   Time|31 minutes
Nutritional Content (per serving)
Cal| 356   Fat| 9g   Protein| 15g   Carbs| 57g   Fiber| 17g

Ingredients:
- Salt (1/4 teaspoon)
- olive oil (2 tablespoons)
- red onion (1/2 cup, chopped)
- red bell pepper (1/3 cup, chopped)
- black beans (1 cup, drained and rinsed)
- Zest and juice (1/2 lime)
- whole wheat tortillas (8, warmed)
- Juice of 1/2 lemon
- trout filets (4, rinsed and dried)
- jicama (1/2 cup, peeled, chopped)
- Fresh cilantro (2/3 cup, finely chopped)
- plain yogurt (1 tablespoon, non-fat)

Directions:
1. Combine your oil, lemon juice and salt.
2. Then pour all of that over the fish fillets and let it marinate for a few minutes.
3. Cook the fish on both side for 3 minutes. In another bowl, combine onion, bell pepper, jicama, cilantro, yogurt and zest and juice of lime to make a salsa.
4. Add your fish on top of a warm tortilla. Top with salsa and fold in half before serving.

Pasta with Turkey and Olives

Servings|4   Time|50 minutes
Nutritional Content (per serving)
Cal| 165   Fat| 4g   Protein| 14g   Carbs| 18g   Fiber| 3g

Ingredients:

- whole wheat pasta (1 pound, uncooked)
- onion (1 Large, peeled, chopped finely)
- turkey breast (1 pound, cut into chunks)
- rosemary (1 teaspoon, dried)
- green bell pepper (1 med, seeded and chopped)
- chicken broth (1 can)
- olive oil (2 teaspoons)
- cloves garlic (4, peeled, finely chopped)
- basil (1 teaspoon, dried)
- black olives (12 med, pitted)
- tomatoes (1 (14 ounces) can, seedless, chopped)
- Romano cheese (1/2 cup, shredded)

Directions:

1. Bring a salted water to boil in a large pot. Add pasta and cook until al dente follow instruction according to the package.
2. While pasta cooks, heat the oil in a large pan over medium heat. Add the garlic and onion. Cook for 6 minutes.
3. Add the turkey, rosemary and basil. Cook for about 8 minutes.
4. Stir in the olives, tomatoes and green pepper and cook for 2 minutes. In the pan add the chicken broth, heat the pan to a boil.
5. Reduce half of the liquid by boiling for 7 minutes. When pasta is done, add to sauce mixture.
6. Toss until pasta is evenly mixed with sauce. Top with cheese and serve.

Pasta with Escarole, Beans and Turkey

Servings|4   Time|36 minutes
Nutritional Content (per serving)
Cal| 289   Fat| 6g   Protein| 24g   Carbs| 36g   Fiber| 16g

Ingredients:

- whole-wheat bowtie pasta (3/4 pound)
- onion (1/2 Medium, chopped)
- turkey (6 ounces, Ground)
- cannellini beans (1(14ounces) can, drained and rinsed)
- chicken broth (1 1/2 cups)
- salt (1/2 teaspoon)
- olive oil (1 tablespoon)
- cloves garlic (3, minced)
- head escarole
- (1 Medium, rinsed, drained and chopped)
- rosemary (1 tablespoon, chopped)
- Parmesan cheese (1/4 cup, grated)

Directions:

1. Bring a salted water to boil in a pot. Add the pasta and follow the cooking instruction on the package.
2. Drain. In a large non-stick pan, heat olive oil over medium heat.
3. Add onion and cook until softened, add garlic and turkey and cook until it browns, about 5 minutes.
4. Add the escarole and cook it for 4 minutes. Add the beans, 1 cup of turkey stock, rosemary, and salt.
5. Simmer until the mixture is slightly thickened. Add the pasta and toss well, thin the sauce with the additional 1/2 cup stock if needed.
6. Top with parmesan cheese. Serve.

Rice Bowl with Shrimp and Peas

Servings|4 Time|1 hour 3 minutes
Nutritional Content (per serving)
Cal| 143   Fat| 4g   Protein| 7g   Carbs| 19g   Fiber| 2g

Ingredients:

- long-grain brown rice (1 cup)
- fresh lemon juice (1/4 cup)
- honey (2 tablespoons)
- shrimp (1 pound, medium, cleaned, peeled, deveined)
- piece fresh ginger (1 (1-inch long) shredded)

- soy sauce (1/4 cup)
- rice vinegar (2 tablespoons)
- olive oil (1 tablespoon)
- snow peas (8 ounces, thawed if frozen, cut in halves)
- Hass avocado (1, chopped)

Directions:

1. Boil 2 cups of water in a saucepan. Add the rice and cover and turn the heat down to simmer.
2. Cook the rice for about 35-45 minutes. In a bowl, fully combine soy sauce, lemon juice, honey, and vinegar.
3. Set your olive oil to get hot on Medium heat in a non-stick pan.
4. Add in your shrimp, ginger and peas then cook for about 3 minutes (or until shrimp becomes pink).
5. Transfer rice to serving bowls, then top with avocado and shrimp mixture. Serve the sauce on the side.

Roasted Chicken and Vegetables

Servings|3   Time|1 hour 10 minutes
Nutritional Content (per serving)
Cal| 147   Fat| 11g   Protein| 2g   Carbs| 13g   Fiber| 3g

Ingredients:

- Roma tomatoes (6, seedless, quartered)
- Potatoes (2 large, unpeeled, quartered)
- cloves garlic (4, finely minced)
- Fresh thyme (1 tablespoon, leaves taken off sprig)
- chicken breast halves (4, skinless)
- Zucchinis (3 medium, chopped coarsely)
- olive oil (3 tablespoons, divided)
- salt (3/4 teaspoon, divided)
- Fresh rosemary (1 tablespoon, chopped)
- lemon zest (1 teaspoon)
- lemon juice (1 tablespoon)

Directions:

1. Preheat oven to 375 degrees F. Put tomatoes, Zucchini and potatoes in a roasting pan, and toss with 2 tablespoons of oil and 1/4 teaspoon salt.
2. Combine lemon zest, thyme, rosemary, garlic, oil, salt and lemon juice. Pour this mixture over chicken.
3. Place chicken in pan with vegetables. Bake in oven for 30 minutes.
4. Stir chicken and vegetables and bake another 25 minutes, or until chicken is cooked through and vegetables are tender.

Shrimp and Black Bean Nachos

Servings|34   Time|25 minutes
Nutritional Content (per serving)
Cal| 172   Fat| 14g   Protein| 4g   Carbs| 12g   Fiber| 5g

Ingredients:

- cilantro (3/4 cup, Fresh chopped)
- lime juice (2 tablespoons)
- Worcestershire sauce (1 teaspoon)
- shrimp (3/4 pound Medium, peeled, cooked, and chopped)
- black bean (1 (15 ounces) can, rinsed and drained)
- red onion (1/2 cup, diced)
- olive oil (1 tablespoon)
- salt (1/2 teaspoon)
- tomatoes (2 cups, seeded, diced)
- avocado (1/2 cup, diced)
- Ground cumin (1/2 teaspoon)
- baked tortilla chips (4 cup)

Directions:

1. In a bowl combine cilantro, onion, lime juice, oil, Worcestershire sauce, shrimp and salt. Cover and refrigerate for 30 minutes.
2. Add tomato and avocado; stir well. Place the cumin and beans in a food processor, and process until smooth.
3. Spread 1-teaspoon black-bean mixture on each chip. Top with 1-tablespoon shrimp mixture. Serve.

Southwestern Chicken Pitas

Servings|6 Time|15 minutes
Nutritional Content (per serving)
Cal| 345 Fat| 12g Protein| 35g Carbs| 22g Fiber| 5g

Ingredients:

- black beans (1 (15 ounces) can, drained, rinsed)
- fresh lime juice (3 tablespoons)
- canola oil (2 tablespoons)
- round whole wheat pita bread (4)
- low-fat provolone cheese (6 slices, cut in halves)
- red bell pepper (1/2 cup, chopped, seeded)
- Fresh cilantro leaves (2 tablespoons, mince)
- chicken breasts (4, boneless, halved, skinless)

Directions:

1. In a bowl, combine beans, bell pepper, lime juice, and cilantro. Set aside. In a pan, heat up the oil over medium heat.
2. Cook chicken in pan until golden brown. Set aside for 10 without cutting. Warm pita bread in oven.
3. Cut chicken into slices. Place half a slice of cheese in center of one pita bread.
4. Top off the sandwich with bean mixture the chicken breast slices. Roll up tightly. Cut in half and serve.

Spaghetti with Zucchini

Servings|4   Time|22 minutes
Nutritional Content (per serving)
Cal| 156   Fat| 11g   Protein| 5g   Carbs| 11g   Fiber| 2g

Ingredients:

- ❖ whole wheat spaghetti (1 pound)
- ❖ butter (2 tablespoons)
- ❖ olive oil (1 tablespoon)
- ❖ Parmesan cheese (1/2 cup, Freshly grated)
- ❖ Zucchinis (2 Medium, grated, water, squeezed out)
- ❖ cloves garlic (2, minced)

Directions:

1. Bring a salted water to boil in a pot. Add pasta and cook until it is al dente or follow the instructions on the package.
2. While pasta cooks, in a large non-stick pan, heat the oil and butter together. Add in the Zucchini and allow cook for 3 minutes.
3. Add in your garlic and continue to cook for another minute, stirring constantly. Add in a half of your parmesan cheese.
4. Transfer past to a serving bowl. Add your Zucchini mixture. Toss then garnish with remaining parmesan cheese. Enjoy!

Summer Spaghetti

Servings|4   Time|23 minutes
Nutritional Content (per serving)
Cal| 548   Fat| 57g   Protein| 3g   Carbs| 14g   Fiber| 3g

Ingredients:

- whole wheat spaghetti (1 pound)
- shallot (1, minced)
- Zucchini (1 medium, chopped)
- green beans (1/2 pound, ends cut)
- basil (1/4 cup, coarsely chopped)
- lemon (1/2 medium, juiced)
- freshly grated lemon peel
- olive oil (1/4 cup)
- cloves garlic (2, minced)
- summer squash (1 medium, chopped)
- salt (1/2 teaspoon)
- unsalted butter (2 tablespoons, room temperature)

Directions:

1. Bring a salted water to boil in a pot. Add pasta and cook until it is al dente or follow the instructions on the package.
2. Heat up the oil over medium heat in a large pan. Add in your garlic and shallot, then stir frequently until fragrant (about 2 minutes).
3. Add the Zucchini, squash, green beans, and basil. Continue to cook, stir occasionally, until all vegetables are tender.
4. Season vegetables with salt and lemon juice. In a large shallow pasta bowl, immediately place the sautéed vegetables with all their juices.
5. Add the butter and linguine, toss to mix well and serve immediately.

White Bean Tortellini

Servings|4   Time|53 minutes
Nutritional Content (per serving)
Cal| 489   Fat| 10g   Protein| 33g   Carbs| 68g   Fiber| 17g

Ingredients:
- olive oil (2 tablespoons)
- onion (1 small, chopped)
- tomatoes (1 cup, seeded and chopped)
- chicken broth (7 cups)
- tortellini (1 pound, with the filling of your choice)
- white beans (2 cups, uncooked)
- garlic cloves (2, finely chopped)
- tomato paste (2 tablespoons)
- bay leaf (1)
- Fresh basil (¼ cup, chopped)

Directions:
1. Soak the beans in water for 8 hours. Drain the beans once you are ready to us it. Heat up the olive oil over medium heat.
2. Add the onion and let it cook for 3 minutes. Mix in the garlic and cook for another minute.
3. Add the tomatoes and tomato paste, stir and cook for a few minutes.
4. Add beans, chicken broth, and bay leaf then allow to boil. Once boiling, lower heat then allow to simmer, without the cover, for another hour and a half.
5. Transfer your mixture to your blender and process into a puree.
6. Adjust the consistency with more stock if necessary.
7. Set a large pot on with salted water and allow to boil. Add in your tortellini and cook as directed by the package.
8. Serve by topping with sauce and basil. Enjoy.

Pink Salmon Cakes & Potatoes

Servings|4   Time|36 minutes
Nutritional Content (per serving)
Cal| 432   Fat| 34g   Protein| 6g   Carbs| 29g   Fiber| 2g

Ingredients:

For Pink salmon Cakes
- ❖ canola oil (3 tablespoons)
- ❖ pink salmon fish (2 (6 ounces) cans, drained)
- ❖ egg (1, beaten)
- ❖ Scallions (2 tablespoons, diced)
- ❖ mayonnaise (1/4 cup, non-fat)
- ❖ whole wheat bread (1/2 cup, cut into small pieces)

For Smashed Potatoes
- ❖ Potatoes (2 large, unpeeled, chopped)
- ❖ salt (2 teaspoons)
- ❖ low fat milk (1/2 cup)
- ❖ unsalted butter (3 tablespoons)

Directions:
1. Cook potatoes in a small saucepan until tender. Drain.
2. Place potatoes back in pan. Heat the butter and milk in microwave until hot.
3. Roughly smash the potatoes with a potato smasher while adding hot liquid until combined and set aside.
4. Combine egg, pink salmon, lemon juice, scallions, mayonnaise, breadcrumbs, and egg in a bowl.
5. Form into patties. Allow to refrigerate and become firm for 10 minutes.
6. Heat oil over medium heat, cook patties until golden brown, about 2 minutes on each side. Serve with potatoes.

Turkey and Barley Casserole

Servings|4 Time|25 minutes
Nutritional Content (per serving)
Cal| 361   Fat| 11g   Protein| 30g   Carbs| 42g   Fiber| 10g

Ingredients:

- Ground turkey (3/4 pound)
- onion (1, chopped finely)
- stalks celery (2, chopped)
- salt (1/2 teaspoon)
- chicken stock (2 1/2 cups)
- poultry seasoning (1 teaspoon)
- carrots (2, chopped)
- green bell pepper (1, seeded and chopped)
- button mushrooms (12, quartered)
- barley (1 cup)
- bay leaf (1)

Directions:

1. Preheat oven to 375 degrees F. Over medium heat, cook Ground turkey with salt until browned, about 5 minutes, in a pan.
2. Add green peppers, celery, carrots and onions. Cook until tender, about 5 minutes.
3. Add bay leaf, poultry seasoning, barley, stock and mushrooms.
4. Mix together and place the mixture in a baking dish. Cover and bake in the preheated oven for 1 hour. Serve.

Lemon Chicken

Servings|4   Time|20 minutes
Nutritional Content (per serving)
Cal| 184   Fat| 9g   Protein| 9g   Carbs| 15g   Fiber| 2g

Ingredients:

- whole wheat pasta (1 pound)
- onion (1 medium, chopped)
- whole wheat flour (2 tablespoons)
- lemon juice (1/4 cup)
- Italian parsley (1/4 cup Fresh, chopped)
- olive oil (2 teaspoons)
- Dijon mustard (1 tablespoon)
- chicken broth (2 cups)
- peas (12 ounces, frozen and thawed)
- chicken (12 ounces cooked, chopped)

Directions:

1. Bring a salted water to boil in a pot. Add and cook the pasta according to the package.
2. Set your olive oil in a non-stick pan to get hot on Medium heat. Stir in the onion and cook for 3 minutes.
3. Stir in your flour and Dijon mustard. Slowly add in your chicken broth while whisking to avoid clumps.
4. Bring the broth to a boil and stir in the lemon juice, parsley, and peas. Add the cooked pasta and chicken to the sauce and serve.

Cucumber Peach Salad

Servings|4 Time|30 minutes
Nutritional Content (per serving)
Cal| 182   Fat| 11g   Protein| 6g   Carbs| 23g   Fiber| 3g

Ingredients:

- Avocados (2 Large, pitted and diced)
- Gala pear (1, unpeeled, cored and diced)
- English cucumber (1, chopped)
- Fresh mint (1/4 cup, chopped)
- Peach (1, unpeeled, pitted and diced)
- Cantaloupe (1 cup, chopped)
- Shallot (1, chopped finely)
- Fresh lime juice (1/4 cup)
- Large lettuce leaves

Directions:

1. In a medium bowl, combine all ingredients except the lettuce leaves. Sprinkle the mint and lime juice.
2. Toss until combine. Let salad sit at least 10-20 minutes. Serve over 2 leaves of lettuce per serving.

String bean Potato Salad

Servings|4-6 Time|22 minutes
Nutritional Content (per serving)
Cal| 142   Fat| 11g   Protein| 1g   Carbs| 10g   Fiber| 1g

Ingredients:

- string beans (1 1/2 pounds, slender)
- red onion (1 small, thinly sliced lengthwise)
- rice vinegar (1/4 cup)
- sugar (1 teaspoon)
- red potatoes (6 small, unpeeled, cubed)
- extra virgin olive oil (1/3 cup)
- garlic salt (1 tablespoon)

Directions:

1. In a pot of boiling water, cook potatoes and string beans about 7 minutes.
2. Drain the contents and run cold water on the beans only to stop cooking process. Drain and set it aside.
3. In a large salad bowl, combine beans, potatoes and onions. For dressing, in a bowl, whisk together olive oil, vinegars, garlic salt and sugar.
4. Toss the vegetables and dressing together until coated. Refrigerate one hour prior to serving.

Bean and Tomato Salad

Servings|4   Time|10 minutes
Nutritional Content (per serving)
Cal| 201   Fat| 14g   Protein| 4g   Carbs| 18g   Fiber| 4g

Ingredients:

- ❖ Tomatoes (4 Medium, seeded and chopped)
- ❖ red onions (1/4 cup, chopped finely)
- ❖ lemon Juice (2 tablespoons)
- ❖ extra virgin olive oil (1/4 cup)
- ❖ garbanzos (2 (14 ounces) cans, drained and rinsed
- ❖ Italian parsley (1 cup, chopped finely)
- ❖ salt (1/2 teaspoon)

Directions:

1. Combine your parsley, onions, beans and tomato. Set aside. In another bowl whisk together salt, olive oil and lemon juice.
2. Pour dressing over vegetables. Mix and serve.

Ricotta & Cannellini Salad

Servings|6   Time|15 minutes
Nutritional Content (per serving)
Cal| 160   Fat| 11g   Protein| 6g   Carbs| 10g   Fiber| 2g

Ingredients:

- plain yogurt (2 tablespoons, low fat)
- fresh lemon juice (2 tablespoons)
- Fresh mint (1 tablespoon, shredded)
- red onions (1/2 cup, thinly sliced)
- tomatoes (3 Medium, seeded and chopped)
- spinach leaves (2 cups)
- extra virgin olive oil (3 tablespoons)
- oregano (3/4 teaspoon, ground)
- white cannellini beans (2 (14 ounces) cans, drained and rinsed)
- Greek olives (1/4 cup, pitted)
- ricotta cheese (1/2 cup, crumbled)

Directions:

1. In a large bowl, combine yogurt, olive oil, lemon juice, oregano, and mint; whisk well.
2. Add onion, beans, tomato, ricotta cheese and olives; toss lightly.
3. Refrigerate for at least one hour. Serve on a bed of spinach.

Bean & Crayfish Salad

Servings|6 Time|20 minutes
Nutritional Content (per serving)
Cal| 334   Fat| 34g   Protein| 3g   Carbs| 7g   Fiber| 3g

Ingredients:

- ❖ Crayfish (1 1/2 pounds, large, cleaned, de-veined and peeled)
- ❖ salt (1/2 teaspoon)
- ❖ fresh Italian parsley (1 tablespoon, chopped)
- ❖ cannellini beans (2 (14 ounces) cans, drained and rinsed)
- ❖ olive oil (1/2 cup)
- ❖ garlic (2 cloves, minced)
- ❖ shallots (2, minced)
- ❖ Fresh sage leaves (1 1/2 tablespoons, chopped)
- ❖ red wine vinegar (1 tablespoon)

Directions:

1. In a glass dish, combine 1/4 teaspoon of salt, garlic and 1/4 cup of the olive oil. Add the crayfish and mix well. Set aside.
2. In a medium bowl, combine the shallots with the remaining 1/4 cup oil and 1/4 teaspoon salt, parsley, sage, and vinegar.
3. Gently stir in the beans. Grill the crayfish over medium heat, turning once, about 3-5 minutes.
4. Serve the crayfish with the bean salad.

Tropical Black Bean Salad

Servings|6 Time|15 minutes
Nutritional Content (per serving)
Cal| 526   Fat| 7g   Protein| 29g   Carbs| 91g   Fiber| 21g

Ingredients:

- ❖ black beans (2 (14 ounces) cans, drained and rinsed)
- ❖ Fresh Italian parsley (1 cup, minced)
- ❖ red bell peppers (2 Medium, seeded and diced)
- ❖ salt (1/4 teaspoon)
- ❖ mangoes (4 Medium, peeled and diced)
- ❖ Scallions (2 Small, chopped finely)
- ❖ extra virgin olive oil (2 tablespoons)
- ❖ balsamic vinegar (1/2 cup)

Directions:

1. In a large salad bowl, combine beans with mangoes, parsley, scallions, and red bell peppers.
2. In a separate Small bowl, whisk together the oil, vinegar and salt. Pour over vegetables and mix well. Serve.

Phase: 1- Meal Plan

Day 1:

Breakfast:
Grape Gelatin
Apple Juice
Simple Black Tea

Mid-Morning Snack:
Cranberry Juice
Cinnamon Gelatin

Lunch:
Carrot & Orange Juice
Water
Chicken Bone & Veggie Broth
Peach Gelatin

Afternoon Snack:
Lemonade
Lemony Black Coffee

Dinner:
Grapes Juice
Veggie Broth
Lemon Gelatin
Lemony Black Tea

Day 2:

Breakfast:
Grape Gelatin
Carrot & Orange Juice
Simple Black Tea

Mid-Morning Snack:
Cranberry Juice
Peach Gelatin

Lunch:
Citrus Apple Juice
Water
Chicken Bones Broth
Cinnamon Gelatin

Afternoon Snack:
Fruit Punch
Citrus Green Tea

Dinner:
Lemony Grapes Juice
Veggie Broth
Lemon Gelatin
Simple Black Tea

Day 3:

Breakfast:
Grapefruit Gelatin
Citrus Apple Juice
Lemony Black Tea

Mid-Morning Snack:
Lemony Grape Juice
Apple Gelatin

Lunch:
Strawberry Juice
Water
Chicken & Veggie Broth
Tangerine Gelatin

Afternoon Snack:
Fruit Punch
Chilled Green Tea

Dinner:
Apple Juice
Fish Broth
Lemon Gelatin
Simple Black Tea

Day 4:

Breakfast:
Cinnamon Gelatin
Grapes Juice
Lemony Black Tea

Mid-Morning Snack:
Cranberry Juice
Lemon Gelatin

Lunch:
Apple Juice
Water
Chicken Bones & Veggie Broth
Peach Gelatin

Afternoon Snack:
Orange, Lemon & Lime Sports Drink
Citrus Green Tea

Dinner:
Strawberry Juice
Veggie Broth
Cinnamon Gelatin
Lemony Black Coffee

Day 5:

Breakfast:
Peach Gelatin
Grapes Juice
Lemony Black Tea

Mid-Morning Snack:
Apple Juice
Grapefruit Gelatin

Lunch:
Orange Juice
Water
Fish & Veggie Broth
Lemon Gelatin

Afternoon Snack:
Apple & Lime Sports Drink
Chilled Green Tea

Dinner:
Strawberry Juice
Chicken Bone Broth
Tangerine Gelatin
Simple Black Tea

Day 6:

Breakfast:
Grapefruit Gelatin
Grapes & Apple Juice
Black Tea

Mid-Morning Snack:
Orange Juice
Lemony Black Coffee

Lunch:
Cranberry Juice
Water
Fish Broth
Apple Gelatin

Afternoon Snack:
Orange, Lemon & Lime Sports Drink
Simple Black Tea

Dinner:
Grapes & Apple Juice
Chicken & Veggie Broth
Lemon Gelatin
Citrus Green Tea

Day 7:

Breakfast:
Tangerine Gelatin
Citrus Apple Juice
Lemony Black Tea

Mid-Morning Snack:
Orange Juice
Cinnamon Gelatin

Lunch:
Lemony Grapes Juice
Water
Veggie Broth
Peach Gelatin

Afternoon Snack:
Mixed Fruit Punch
Chilled Green Tea

Dinner:
Strawberry Juice
Fish & Veggie Broth
Lemon Gelatin
Citrus Green Tea

Phase: 2- Meal Plan

Day 1:

Breakfast:
Vanilla Waffles

Lunch:
Beet Soup

Dinner:
Prawn with Asparagus

Day 2:

Breakfast:
Chicken & Veggie Muffins

Lunch:
Cucumber & Yogurt Salad

Dinner:
Chicken with Bell peppers

Day 3:

Breakfast:
Pumpkin Pancakes

Lunch:
Pasta with Asparagus

Dinner:
Salmon Salad

Day 4:

Breakfast:
Green Veggies Quiche

Lunch:
Chicken & Carrot Wraps

Dinner:
Pasta Soup

Day 5:

Breakfast:
Tomato & Basil Scramble

Lunch:
Mushroom Curry

Dinner:

Day 6:

Breakfast:
Zucchini Bread

Lunch:
Tuna Stuffed Avocado

Dinner:
Scallops with Spinach

Day 7:

Breakfast:
Carrot, Tomato & Celery Juice

Lunch:
Squash Mac 'n Cheese

Dinner:
Seafood Stew

Phase: 3- Meal Plan

Day 1:

Breakfast:
Pumpkin Oatmeal

Lunch:
Beans & Olives Enchiladas

Dinner:
Pasta with Quinoa Sauce

Day 2:

Breakfast:
Eggless Veggie Omelet

Lunch:
Fruit, Avocado & Cucumber Salad

Dinner:
Beans & Sweet Potato Soup

Day 3:

Breakfast:
Bulgur Porridge

Lunch:
Chickpea Balls in Tomato Sauce

Dinner:
Turkey & Lentil Soup

Day 4:

Breakfast:
Savory Crepes

Lunch:
Quinoa, Beans & Mango Salad

Dinner:
Rice, Lentil & Veggie Casserole

Day 5:

Breakfast:
Oats & Quinoa Porridge

Lunch:
Farro & Veggies Salad

Dinner:
Three Beans Chili

Day 6:

Breakfast:
Apple & Banana Porridge

Lunch:
Lentils with Kale

Dinner:
Pasta & Chickpeas Curry

Day 7:

Breakfast:
Spinach & Avocado Smoothie Bowl

Lunch:
Chickpeas Stuffed Avocado

Dinner:
Turkey & Beans Chili

Index

Printed in Great Britain
by Amazon